Postanesthesia Care Unit

Guest Editor

SCOTT A. FALK, MD

ANESTHESIOLOGY CLINICS

www.anesthesiology.theclinics.com

Consulting Editor
LEE A. FLEISHER, MD, FACC

September 2012 • Volume 30 • Number 3

SAUNDERS an imprint of ELSEVIER, Inc.

W.B. SAUNDERS COMPANY
A Division of Elsevier Inc.

1600 John F. Kennedy Boulevard, Suite 1800 ● Philadelphia, PA 19103-2899

http://www.theclinics.com

ANESTHESIOLOGY CLINICS Volume 30, Number 3
September 2012 ISSN 1932-2275, ISBN-13: 978-1-4557-4209-7

Editor: Pamela Hetherington

Anesthesiology Clinics (ISSN 1932-2275) is published quarterly by Elsevier Inc., 360 Park Avenue South, New York, NY 10010-1710. Months of issue are March, June, September, and December. Periodicals postage paid at New York, NY and at additional mailing offices. Subscription prices are $154.00 per year (US student/resident), $313.00 per year (US individuals), $383.00 per year (Canadian individuals), $496.00 per year (US institutions), $615.00 per year (Canadian institutions), $216.00 per year (Canadian and foreign student/resident), $434.00 per year (foreign individuals), and $615.00 per year (foreign institutions). To receive student and resident rate, orders must be accompanied by name of affiliated institution, date of term, and the *signature* of program/residency coordinator on institutions letterhead. Orders will be billed at individual rate until proof of status is received. Foreign air speed delivery is included in all *Clinics'* subscription prices. All prices are subject to change without notice. POSTMASTER: Send address changes to *Anesthesiology Clinics,* Elsevier Health Sciences Division, Subscription Customer Service, 3251 Riverport Lane, Maryland Heights, MO 63043. Customer Service (orders, claims, online, change of address): Elsevier Health Sciences Division, Subscription Customer Service, 3251 Riverport Lane, Maryland Heights, MO 63043. Tel:1-800-654-2452 (U.S. and Canada); 314-447-8871 (outside U.S. and Canada). Fax: 314-447-8029. E-mail: journalscustomerservice-usa@elsevier.com (for print support); journalsonlinesupport-usa@elsevier.com (for online support).

Reprints. For copies of 100 or more of articles in this publication, please contact the Commercial Reprints Department, Elsevier Inc., 360 Park Avenue South, New York, NY 10010-1710. Tel.: 212-633-3812; Fax: 212-462-1935; E-mail: reprints@elsevier.com.

Anesthesiology Clinics, is also published in Spanish by McGraw-Hill Inter-americana Editores S. A., P.O. Box 5-237, 06500 Mexico D. F., Mexico.

Anesthesiology Clinics, is covered in *MEDLINE/PubMed (Index Medicus), Current Contents/Clinical Medicine, Excerpta Medica, ISI/BIOMED,* and *Chemical Abstracts.*

Printed and bound by CPI Group (UK) Ltd, Croydon, CR0 4YY

Transferred to Digital Print 2012

Contributors

CONSULTING EDITOR

LEE A. FLEISHER, MD, FACC
Robert D. Dripps Professor and Chair of Anesthesiology and Critical Care, Perelman School of Medicine, University of Pennsylvania, Philadelphia, Pennsylvania

GUEST EDITOR

SCOTT A. FALK, MD
Assistant Professor of Anesthesiology and Critical Care, Medical Director PACU, Hospital of the University of Pennsylvania; Department of Anesthesiology and Critical Care, Perelman School of Medicine, University of Pennsylvania, Philadelphia, Pennsylvania

AUTHORS

KARA BETH CHENITZ, MD
Fellow, Renal, Electrolyte and Hypertension Division, Department of Internal Medicine, Hospital of the University of Pennsylvania, Philadelphia, Pennsylvania

JASON CWIK, MD
Chair, Department of Anesthesiology and Critical Care, Pennsylvania Hospital, Philadelphia, Pennsylvania

LEOPOLD H.J. EBERHART, MD, PhD, MA
Department of Anaesthesiology and Intensive Care, Philipps-University Marburg, Marburg, Germany

SCOTT A. FALK, MD
Assistant Professor of Anesthesiology and Critical Care, Medical Director PACU, Hospital of the University of Pennsylvania; Department of Anesthesiology and Critical Care, Perelman School of Medicine, University of Pennsylvania, Philadelphia, Pennsylvania

NICOLE HOKE, MSN, RN, CCRN, CCNS
PACU Clinical Nurse Specialist, Hospital of the University of Pennsylvania, Philadelphia, Pennsylvania

W. SCOTT JELLISH, MD, PhD
Professor and Chairman, Department of Anesthesiology, Loyola University Medical Center, Maywood, Illinois

JOHANNA JOKINEN
Department of Anaesthesia and Critical Care, University Hospitals of Würzburg, Würzburg, Germany

PETER KRANKE, MD, PhD, MBA
Professor of Anaesthesia, Department of Anaesthesia and Critical Care, University Hospitals of Würzburg, Würzburg, Germany

MEGHAN B. LANE-FALL, MD
Clinical Associate and Post-doctoral Research Fellow, Department of Anesthesiology and Critical Care, Hospital of the University of Pennsylvania, Philadelphia, Pennsylvania

RICHARD MORROW, MBA, MBB
Executive Director and Leader, Quality, Safety, Reliability, Healthcare Performance Partners, Nashville, Tennessee

PATRICK J. NELIGAN, MD
Department of Anesthesia & Intensive Care, Galway University Hospitals, Galway, Ireland

MICHAEL O'ROURKE, MD
Assistant Professor, Department of Anesthesiology, Loyola University Medical Center, Maywood, Illinois

ANDREW PLANTE, MD
Clinical Instructor of Anesthesiology, Department of Anesthesiology & Perioperative Medicine, University Hospitals, Case Medical Center, Cleveland, Ohio

ELIOT RO, MD
Assistant Professor of Anesthesiology, PACU Medical Director, Department of Anesthesiology & Perioperative Medicine, University Hospitals, Case Medical Center, Cleveland, Ohio

NORBERT ROEWER, MD, PhD
Professor of Anaesthesia and Chair, Department of Anaesthesia and Critical Care, University Hospitals of Würzburg, Würzburg, Germany

JAMES R. ROWBOTTOM, MD, FCCP
Associate Professor of Anesthesiology and Surgery, Vice Chair of Clinical Affairs, Clinical Director Operative Services, Chief of Perioperative Medicine, Department of Anesthesiology & Perioperative Medicine, University Hospitals, Case Medical Center, Cleveland, Ohio

NICHOLAS RUSSO, MD
Medical Director, Intensive Care Unit, Medina General Hospital, Medina, Ohio; Staff Anesthesiologist/Intensivist, Anesthesia Critical Care Institute, Cleveland Clinic Foundation, Cleveland, Ohio

ANDREW F. SMITH
Consultant Anaesthetist, Director, Lancaster Patient Safety Research Unit, Royal Lancaster Infirmary, Lancaster, United Kingdom

Contents

> Patients in the perioperative and postanesthesia care unit (PACU) experience several transitions in patient care at the same time that the majority of major morbidities will arise. The transitions for these patients are at the critical juncture between surgery and a steady sustained recovery. Historically these important medical problems have been addressed as a nonformalized process. The authors have introduced a formalized process, based on interdisciplinary rounding strategies used in intensive care units, to attend patients and address problems.

> Spinal and epidural anesthesia and analgesia, and the combination of the two techniques, have been excellent choices for the management of certain surgical procedures and continue to grow in popularity. The demand for increased patient mobility and quicker discharge for both inpatients and outpatients lends itself to the benefits of regional anesthesia. A neuraxial block is indicated for any surgical procedure in which the appropriate sensory level can be accomplished without any adverse outcome. This article outlines the indications and contraindications for these techniques.

> Perioperative hyperglycemia has potential significant adverse consequences of increased mortality and morbidity including surgical site infection, renal insufficiency and anemia requiring transfusion. Both diabetic and non-diabetic patients are affected adversely by perioperative hyperglycemia. However, these two subgroups do not necessarily benefit equally from perioperative glycemic control. Moreover, ideal target glucose range as well as the appropriate patient population(s) for whom glycemic control offers the most benefit have yet to be fully elucidated. However, there are clear potential adverse consequences of tight control such as hypoglycemia.

> Postoperative anxiety has received less attention historically than preoperative anxiety. Recognition that anxiety occurs throughout the perioperative period has led to increased interest in identifying and treating

anxiety in the postoperative period. This article outlines the causes of postoperative anxiety, how it is classified, the effects of anxiety on outcomes after surgery, and some of the clinical procedures that produce the highest levels of anxiety for patients. In addition, an attempt is made to delineate the major risk factors for developing postoperative anxiety and the classic therapeutic modalities used to reduce symptoms and treat the psychological manifestations of anxiety.

Johanna Jokinen, Andrew F. Smith, Norbert Roewer, Leopold H.J. Eberhart, and Peter Kranke

Postoperative nausea and vomiting (PONV) constitutes a significant factor in delaying recovery after anesthesia and impairing patient satisfaction. To date the prevention of PONV using single or multimodal interventions, usually based on risk assessment, has gained some popularity. However, comprehensive implementation and knowledge transfer of the latest accomplishments in the prevention of PONV is only slowly being adopted into clinical practice. Preventing PONV is the first step in avoiding refractory PONV. This review comments mainly on the management of refractory PONV. As the data on coping with established PONV are rare, further studies focusing on treatment of established PONV are needed.

Patrick J. Neligan

General anesthesia and surgery are associated with changes in the shape of the chest that result in atelectasis, a major factor in the development of postoperative respiratory failure. Postoperative noninvasive positive pressure ventilation (NIPPV) has been shown to improve oxygenation and ventilation for high-risk patients. NIPPV has been used as rescue therapy for patients developing acute respiratory distress postoperatively, and appears to be most frequently successful in patients whose problem is atelectasis or obesity. Failure to respond to NIPPV after 20 minutes is usually an indication of intubation, mechanical ventilation, and transfer to the intensive care unit.

Kara Beth Chenitz and Meghan B. Lane-Fall

Decreased urine output and acute kidney injury (also known as acute renal failure) are among the most important complications that may develop in the postanesthetic period. In this article, the authors present definitions of decreased urine output, oliguria, and acute kidney injury. They review the epidemiology, pathophysiology, and prevention of postoperative acute kidney injury. Finally, the article offers approaches to diagnosis and management of the postsurgical patient with decreased urine output or acute kidney injury.

Andrew Plante, Eliot Ro, and James R. Rowbottom

The clinician caring for patients in the immediate postoperative period must maintain a high index of suspicion for the development of complications.

Evolving illness manifests itself throughout the continuum of care and must be recognized and aggressively managed to ensure optimal outcome. This article discusses common hemodynamic problems encountered in the postanesthesia care unit. These problems are presented in a clinical framework that is familiar to experienced practitioners and recognizable to trainees. This article reviews of these common problems including relevant physiologic principles; effects on hemodynamics; and a logical approach to evaluation, monitoring, and management of a complex postoperative patient.

Richard Morrow

Health care quality and safety are becoming more transparent, and consumers will increasingly value safety and quality rating in choosing where they go for surgery. Perioperative services are major drivers to a hospital's safety rating. Surgical services are often the most, or one of the most, profitable services, and loss of referrals and poor media reports will directly reduce margins. This article aims to guide leaders and perioperative staff in how to start improving perioperative quality and safety in health care and surgical services.

ANESTHESIOLOGY CLINICS

RELATED INTEREST

Critical Care Clinics, October 2011 (Volume 24, Issue 4)
Venous Thromboembolism in Critical Care
Kenneth Wood, *Guest Editor*

DOWNLOAD
Free App!

Review Articles
THE CLINICS

NOW AVAILABLE FOR YOUR iPhone and iPad

Foreword

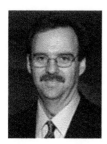

Lee A. Fleisher, MD, FACC
Consulting Editor

In the context of health care reform, it is increasingly important for anesthesiologists to demonstrate their value in patient care. While most anesthesiologists focus on our role in intraoperative care, the Post Anesthesia Care Unit (PACU) is clearly within our domain and improvements in care in this area can significantly impact the entire perioperative experience. This includes strategies to treat medical conditions that arise intra- and post-operatively as well as treatment of postoperative pain. It is increasingly important for anesthesiologists to ensure that pain is well controlled and that the patient transitions to the next phase of care. This importance is highlighted by the inclusion of pain questions in the HCAPS survey. Additionally, techniques developed in the intensive care unit are now being brought into the PACU, such as interdisciplinary rounds and patient- and family-centered postoperative care. In this issue of *Anesthesiology Clinics*, the guest editor has solicited a series of experts to write on these important issues relevant to all anesthesiologists.

In choosing a guest editor for this issue, I solicited Scott A. Falk, MD, Assistant Professor of Clinical Anesthesiology and Critical Care at the University of Pennsylvania Perelman School of Medicine. Scott completed his anesthesiology residency at University Hospitals of Cleveland/CASE School of Medicine, after which he completed a fellowship in critical care medicine at the Cleveland Clinic. After a brief period on the faculty at the CASE School of Medicine, he was recruited to the University of Pennsylvania, where he participates in both intraoperative care and the intensive care unit. For the past several years Scott has been the Medical Director of the PACU and is one of the quality officers of the Department, involved in transformational change in the Hospital of the University of Pennsylvania. After reading the current issue, you will clearly find that he has forward-thinking ideas on how best to transform the anesthesiologist's role in the PACU.

Lee A. Fleisher, MD, FACC
University of Pennsylvania School of Medicine
3400 Spruce Street, Dulles 680
Philadelphia, PA 19104, USA

E-mail address:
lee.fleisher@uphs.upenn.edu

Anesthesiology Clin 30 (2012) ix
http://dx.doi.org/10.1016/j.anclin.2012.08.004   **anesthesiology.theclinics.com**
1932-2275/12/$ – see front matter © 2012 Published by Elsevier Inc.

Preface

Postoperative Care

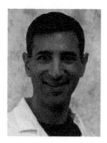

Scott A. Falk, MD
Guest Editor

In the early days of anesthesia and surgery the postoperative or postanesthesia care unit (PACU) was a location in which patients would continue to recover from the lingering effects of anesthesia. As anesthetic care has advanced, this recovery period has evolved to what is essentially a transitional area in which patients receive varying intensity of care as they either begin their recovery and healing process or are triaged to higher level units.

The PACU has different meanings and plays widely varying roles depending on the needs of a particular patient or the population served. At the Hospital of the University of Pennsylvania PACU, we essentially conducted an experiment by assessing daily the most pressing patient needs encountered in the unit. These findings led to the creation of the articles included in this issue.

The first article is a detailed look at the interdisciplinary rounding process in the ICU and the ways in which interdisciplinary rounding have been utilized to improve outcomes in ICU environments. Implementing this "rounding" paradigm is important as PACUs become more than transitional spaces. It implies that they are evolving to become important care areas where healing begins.

The next 2 articles give a detailed look at multimodal pain control as well as neuraxial analgesia in the PACU. Pain control is vital in the perioperative period not only for organic medical reasons, ie., reducing surgical stress responses, but also is a tremendous value-added outcome measure by patients. Early pain control undoubtedly leads to better longer term pain management and patient emotional well-being during the healing process. Common complications of neuraxial analgesia that should be diagnosed in the early postoperative period are addressed.

We found that other common patient-centered problems in the PACU included anxiety and postoperative nausea and vomiting. The articles on these subjects do an excellent job reviewing the current standards of care as well as addressing possible advances that we will see in the near future. Of particular interest were the complementary medicine treatments available for anxiolysis in the perioperative period. Advanced

Anesthesiology Clin 30 (2012) xi–xii
http://dx.doi.org/10.1016/j.anclin.2012.07.013
1932-2275/12/$ – see front matter © 2012 Published by Elsevier Inc.

pharmacologic strategies for treatment of refractory postoperative nausea and vomiting are delineated.

Commonly occurring and vitally important medical problems are addressed in detail. Perioperative hemodynamic dysregulation, treatment, and monitoring modalities are described. Common scenarios with appropriate actions are addressed. Oliguria and perioperative renal injury and dysfunction are addressed. Diagnostic and treatment options for this devastating complication are characterized. The importance of perioperative glycemic control is conveyed. This detailed view of this physiologic derangement gives insight into both causes and treatments of glycemic dysregulation and its importance to healing and well-being. The modality of postoperative noninvasive ventilation is also described. As our population moves toward one with increasing incidence of obesity and obstructive sleep apnea, this will become more essential. As anesthesiologists take care of patients with increasing morbidities, a deep understanding of these medical issues and their implications in the perioperative care period will become essential.

We end this issue by addressing postoperative quality assurance and improvement. Health care, in general, and perioperative services, in particular, are becoming more resource intense and expensive. Ensuring high levels of perioperative quality will be essential in the future as we strive to continue to provide better care more efficiently to our patient population.

I am delighted with the work the authors have contributed to this issue. It is my hope that the future of perioperative care continues to evolve into the essential time of healing.

I would also like to thank Pamela Hetherington for all of her time and patience. I am especially grateful to my family for their love and support. They make it all worthwhile.

Scott A. Falk, MD
Department of Anesthesiology and Critical Care
Perelman School of Medicine
University of Pennsylvania
Philadelphia, PA 19104, USA

E-mail address:
Scott.falk@uphs.upenn.edu

Interdisciplinary Rounds in the Postanesthesia Care Unit

A New Perioperative Paradigm

Nicole Hoke, MSN, RN, CCRN, CCNS[a],*, Scott Falk, MD[a,b]

KEYWORDS

- Postanesthesia care unit • Multidisciplinary rounding • Postoperative morbidity

KEY POINT

- Interdisciplinary rounds in the post anesthesia care unit facilitated improved quality of care, reduced variations in care, and enhanced learning and interaction between physicians, house staff, and nursing staff.

INTRODUCTION

In the postanesthesia care unit (PACU) there has been an identified need to improve interdisciplinary communication between nursing and anesthesia in order to provide seamless care for the postoperative patient. Structured rounding processes can be an effective method to improve communication among health care providers.[1] It has been shown that interdisciplinary rounds have been associated with better patient outcomes, improved efficiency of care, and decreased mortality.[2] Studies and articles related to the advantages of interdisciplinary rounds have been focused on areas outside of the perioperative arena. The authors chose to create a structured rounding process with an interdisciplinary group in the PACU to improve the quality of care for the recovering postoperative patient. This article describes the process one institution used to implement interdisciplinary rounds in the PACU.

Health care institutions are constantly searching for ways to improve patient service, increase efficiency, improve outcomes, and reduce errors. To date there is scant literature published on interdisciplinary rounding in the postanesthesia care environment. Clark[3] demonstrated that patient care rounds by clinical nurses and educators in the postanesthesia care setting increased accountability for nursing practice, which improved the delivery of care to patients. However, this approach was limited because it did not include an interdisciplinary group of health care providers. Most other

[a] Perioperative Nursing, Hospital of the University of Pennsylvania, 3400 Spruce Street, Philadelphia, PA 19104, USA; [b] Perelman School of Medicine, University of Pennsylvania, Philadelphia, PA 19104, USA
* Corresponding author.
E-mail address: Nicole.Hoke@uphs.upenn.edu

Anesthesiology Clin 30 (2012) 427–431
http://dx.doi.org/10.1016/j.anclin.2012.07.008   **anesthesiology.theclinics.com**
1932-2275/12/$ – see front matter © 2012 Elsevier Inc. All rights reserved.

published studies supporting interdisciplinary rounds have been conducted in settings outside of the perioperative arena. A fully integrated approach to interdisciplinary team rounding has been shown to improve communication, reduce nosocomial infections, and improve care efficiency.[4–7] A 2011 study documented a 24% decrease in the rate of ventilator-associated pneumonia more than 1 year after a rounding team adopted a formalized checklist system to address quality issues.[8] A population-based state-wide study in 2010 demonstrated an overall decrease in mortality (odds ratio 0.78) in hospitals using multidisciplinary rounds in the intensive care unit and high-intensity physician staffing.[9]

IMPLEMENTATION

A goal of improving interdisciplinary communication between nursing and anesthesia was identified by the PACU medical director and the PACU clinical nurse specialist. By improving communication the authors hoped to facilitate improved quality of care, reduce variations in care, and enhance learning and interaction between physicians, house staff, and nursing staff. To provide direction for interdisciplinary rounding in the PACU, goals were established, which are shown in **Box 1**. The goals were at the forefront and focus of each rounding session.

In a collaborative effort the authors created an interdisciplinary rounding team to evaluate patients' real time in the PACU. The rounding team was created to increase communication between nursing staff and physicians, improve transitions in care, eliminate variations in care, and establish best practices for the postoperative patient. The rounding team consists of the attending anesthesiologist, a PACU dedicated anesthesia resident, the patients' primary bedside nurse, the PACU clinical nurse specialist, and the PACU charge nurse. Representatives from the pharmacy department and respiratory therapy department are also invited to attend; however, participation varies based on schedule. For the initiation of this system change, rounds were conducted twice a week in the PACU. The process was clearly defined by the group before the initiation rounds. The primary nurse presents the PACU patient by using a rounding tool (**Fig. 1**), which was developed to formalize the care and track the data collected on PACU patients. It also assures that key quality metrics are discussed. During rounds the interdisciplinary group reviews all of the information about the patient including medical history, the operative course, and a systems assessment with the goal of implementing best practices and eliminating variations in care for the patient population.

RESULTS

Since the initiation of interdisciplinary rounds, the authors have currently rounded on 138 patients in the PACU. Through this collaborative process they have improved the

---

Box 1
Goals

1. Improve transitions in care by developing interdisciplinary PACU rounding

2. Eliminate variations in care

3. Establish and implement best practices for perioperative patients

4. Improve patient and family-centered care to provide communication with the patient and family regarding the postoperative plan of care

5. Provide accountability for perfect care for patients in the PACU. Strive for consistent evidence-based care for the postoperative patient

Surgical Procedure: PM/S Hx:

Diagnosis:

Nursing Concerns	Allergies:

INTRAOP	Crystalloid _____ VTE Prophylaxis _____ Colloid _____ Antibiotics _____ Urine _____ __ Medications _____ IUC: Y/N EBL _____ Intra-operative Events: Anesthesia ☐ GETA ☐ G-LMA ☐ SPINAL ☐ EPIDURAL ☐ REGIONAL BLOCK ☐ MAC Muscle Relaxant ☐ YES ☐ NO REVERSED ☐ YES ☐ NO

NEURO	GCS _____ Admission RASS _____ Current RASS _____	**CARDIO VASCULAR**	Temp. _____ HR _____ Rhythm _____ BP _____ Goal BP _____
RESP	O2 requirement _____ Pulse ox _____ Chest Tube/s:	**GI/GU**	PONV _____ Urine _____ Bladder Scan ☐ Y ☐ N Amount _____
SKIN/ DRAINS	Surgical Site _____ Drains :	**PATIENT FAMILY**	
PAIN	Admission Pain Score _____ Current Pain Score _____ Pain Medication _____	**LABS/TESTS**	

PLAN OF CARE	IVF _____ GTTS _____ Antibiotics _____
Interventions	

Fig. 1. PACU rounding tool.

care of the recovering PACU patient at their institution, improved house staff and nursing bedside education, and made several important systems and process changes to increase safety and reliability. Transitions in care have been refined and improved by having a definitive plan of care that the interdisciplinary group can follow in the postoperative phase and provide a seamless transition to the inpatient unit. Staff satisfaction has improved on the unit by having the interdisciplinary group review patient issues arising in the PACU in a timely manner. Rounding has reduced variations in care by presenting staff with case studies from rounds on a monthly basis. Case studies allow for the dissemination of information on the latest trends in caring for the postoperative patient. Since the initiation of rounds, the group has been able to better standardize care for the patient immediately arriving in the PACU. Setting goals for control of blood pressure on arrival in the PACU, eliminating the use of T-pieces in favor of pressure-supported ventilation and creating a process for easier ordering of bronchodilators are 3 examples of changes in systems that have taken place.

This formalized process has also allowed identification of the most pressing problems in the localized PACU setting so that focus can be directed on educational efforts toward the elimination of these problems. Pain management, hemodynamic problems, and respiratory problems accounted for more than 61% of major perioperative concerns (**Fig. 2**). These problems have been addressed on several levels, from individual education to departmental conferences. Having quality control data has allowed the team to track the prevalence and resolution of problems over time.

Historically in the postoperative care unit, family members have not had the opportunity to visit. After identifying this as a major concern for 14% of their population, the authors began to include the patient and family, when available, in rounds in the PACU. This inclusion provided an opportunity to explain to the patient and family the plan of care following discharge from the PACU to home or the inpatient unit.

SPECIFIC CLINICAL VIGNETTES

- A 54-year-old patient scheduled for an exploratory laparotomy and total hysterectomy. Medical history included fibroids, hypertension, and type 2 diabetes. The patient arrived at the PACU in pain, rating it 10/10; location: right lower extremity. The patient was admitted to the PACU postoperatively. The PACU registered nurse admitted the patient and the clinical nurse specialist assessed the patient. Because of the pain level and location, rounds were performed on admission to the PACU. The patient's right lower extremity was pale on assessment and negative for a pedal pulse. The patient was returned to the operating room within 40 minutes for thrombectomy.
- A 68-year-old patient scheduled for bilateral mastectomies and free flap reconstruction. Medical history included sleep apnea, continuous positive airway pressure at home, rheumatoid arthritis, and fibromyalgia. There was delayed awakening in the operating room; the patient remained intubated on arrival at the PACU. The patient arrived on 60% T-piece with a pulse oximetry of 93%,

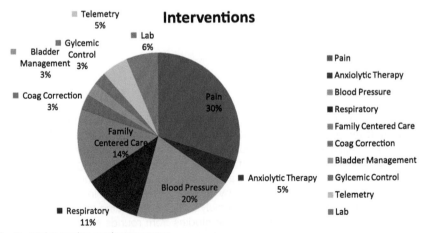

Fig. 2. Major perioperative concerns.

and admission Richmond Agitation Sedation Score of −3. Arterial blood gas: 7.22/68/98/23 → 60% T-piece. The patient placed on a ventilator with pressure support. Use of T-piece was eliminated.

DISCUSSION

Implementation of interdisciplinary rounds was not without its challenges. Providers needed convincing that PACU interdisciplinary rounds was a valuable use of time. An effort was made to expand the providers' prospective that interdisciplinary rounds were beneficial to the overall care of the perioperative patient, and included discussion of the multiple handoffs and transitions in care that occur within the perioperative arena. Staff was able to understand the important impact rounds can have on the plan of care for the perioperative patient. Within the first 6 months of rounding, staff started to express high satisfaction, as a result of which PACU interdisciplinary rounds were increased from twice per week to daily. The authors have improved the care of the recovering PACU patient at their institution through the implementation of PACU interdisciplinary rounds. Through PACU rounds, bedside education has increased and several important changes in systems and processes have been identified to increase safety and reliability. Transitions in care have been refined and improved by having a definitive plan of care that the interdisciplinary group can follow in the postoperative phase and thus provide a seamless transition to the inpatient unit. As one navigates through this new process of rounding in the perioperative arena, it has become evident that the care of the patient is being directly influenced in a positive manner.

REFERENCES

1. Sehgal NL, Auerbach AA. Communication failures and a call for new systems to promote patient safety: comment on "Structured interdisciplinary rounds in a medical teaching unit". Arch Intern Med 2011;171(7):684–5.
2. Plantinga LC, Fink NE, Jaar BG, et al. Frequency of sit-down patient care rounds, attainment of clinical performance targets, hospitalization, and mortality in hemodialysis patients. J Am Soc Nephrol 2004;15(12):3144–53.
3. Clark KL. Nursing patient care rounds in the postanesthesia care unit setting. J Post Anesth Nurs 1994;9(1):20–5.
4. Jain M, Miller L, Belt D, et al. Decline in ICU adverse events, nosocomial infections and cost through a quality improvement initiative focusing on teamwork and culture change. Qual Saf Health Care 2006;15(4):235–9.
5. Dutton RP, Cooper C, Jones A, et al. Daily multidisciplinary rounds shorten length of stay for trauma patients. J Trauma 2003;55(5):913–9.
6. Vazirani S, Hays RD, Shapiro MF, et al. Effect of a multidisciplinary intervention on communication and collaboration among physicians and nurses. Am J Crit Care 2005;14(1):71–7.
7. Halm MA, Gagner S, Goering MM, et al. Interdisciplinary rounds: impact on patients, families, and staff. Clin Nurse Spec 2003;17(3):133–42.
8. Dubose J, Teixeira PG, Inaba K, et al. Measurable outcomes of quality improvement using a daily quality rounds checklist: one-year analysis in a trauma intensive care unit with sustained ventilator-associated pneumonia reduction. J Trauma 2010;69(4):855–60.
9. Kim MM, Barnato AE, Angus DC, et al. The effect of multidisciplinary care teams on intensive care unit mortality. Arch Intern Med 2010;170(4):369–76.

Postoperative Considerations of Neuraxial Anesthesia

Jason Cwik, MD

KEYWORDS

- Neuraxial anesthesia • Cardiovascular effects • Dermatomal levels
- Postoperative hypercoagulability

KEY POINTS

- A neuraxial block is indicated for any surgical procedure in which the appropriate sensory level can be accomplished without any adverse patient outcomes.
- When choosing the neuraxial technique: consider the length of the procedure, whether there is a need for postoperative analgesia, and what is most appropriate for the patient's condition.
- Local anesthetics alone or in combination with opioids are commonly used for postoperative infusions either epidurally or intrathecally.

Spinal and epidural anesthesia and analgesia, and the combination of the two techniques, combined spinal epidural (CSE), have been excellent choices for the management of certain surgical procedures and continue to grow in popularity. The demand for increased patient mobility and quicker discharge for both inpatients and outpatients lends itself to the benefits of regional anesthesia. A neuraxial block is indicated for any surgical procedure in which the appropriate sensory level can be accomplished without any adverse patient outcomes.

Preoperatively, the patient must undergo all the appropriate preparations regardless of the choice of the anesthesia technique that is ultimately chosen. The final determination for the selection of the regional anesthesia technique is the suitability of the patient for the technique. Patient selection must take into account physical characteristics, pathophysiology, and psychological states (**Box 1**).[1]

Despite the many similarities of spinal and epidural anesthesia in the placement and the resultant sensory, motor, and sympathetic blockade, there are many differences. Spinal anesthesia uses very small doses that may have a profound effect on some systems but has very little systemic pharmacologic effect. In contrast, epidural anesthetic doses are typically larger and may cause a systemic pharmacologic effect. These similarities and differences of spinal and epidural anesthesia lend themselves

Department of Anesthesiology and Critical Care, Pennsylvania Hospital, 800 Spruce Street, Philadelphia, PA 19107, USA
E-mail address: jason.cwik@uphs.upenn.edu

Anesthesiology Clin 30 (2012) 433–443
http://dx.doi.org/10.1016/j.anclin.2012.07.005
1932-2275/12/$ – see front matter © 2012 Elsevier Inc. All rights reserved.

> **Box 1**
> **Contraindications against central neuraxial blockade**
>
> *Absolute*
> - Fulminant sepsis
> - Massive site infection
> - Severe hypovolemia or hypotension
> - Coagulopathy
>
> *Relative*
> - Neuropathy
> - Neurologic or demyelinating disease
> - Some cardiac dysfunctions and diseases (severe aortic stenosis)
> - Unwilling patient
> - Uncertain surgical procedure

to a wide range of flexibility while taking care of a patient. When deciding which neuraxial block, or combined technique, to use, many factors should be considered.

Factors to consider when choosing the neuraxial technique include:

1. Length of procedure: do not want to wait for an epidural to take effect. If length cannot be accurately determined, a CSE technique may work best.
2. Determine if there is a need for postoperative analgesia.
3. If there is no clear procedure reason, do what is most appropriate for the patient's condition, taking into account medical needs and the discharge indications for the patient.

PHYSIOLOGIC EFFECTS OF NEURAXIAL ANESTHESIA

The physiologic effects of spinal and epidural anesthesia will depend on many factors, such as the dermatomal level, the amount of drug injected, and the level that it was injected. The interruption of spinal cord function begins caudally and proceeds in the cephalad direction. Autonomic function is lost before sensory function, which is lost, in turn, before motor function.

Neural blockade requires the blockage of the sodium channel after the diffusion through the lipid membrane. Nerve fibers are not homogeneous and consist of three main fiber types: A, B, and C. Because of the mixture of the fiber types, onset is not the same from person to person and level to level. The motor fibers are the most heavily myelinated and will require the highest drug concentration for blockade, their function will also be the first to return. The level of the autonomic block will be approximately two dermatomal levels above the skin analgesic level, which is two dermatomal levels above the motor blockade. This becomes important for the surgical level needed and when evaluating the level depending on which modality is being assessed: sympathetic, sensory, or motor.[2]

CARDIOVASCULAR EFFECTS

The sympathetic nervous system is blocked in proportion to the height of the anesthesia level obtained. The sympathetic chain arises from the thoracic and lumbar spinal cord; these innervate the smooth muscle of the arterial and venous circulation.

The arterial circulation retains most of its tone but this is not true of the venous circulation. The loss of tone in the venous circulation will create pooling and a subsequent decrease in venous return. Heart rate is partially controlled by the sympathetic afferents to the heart (T1–T4) and may be blocked by either spinal or epidural blockade; this would result in unopposed vagal tone and bradycardia.

The degree of hypotension that may occur from sympathetic blockade will be determined by the amount of dermatomal levels that are blocked. Treatment will consist of increasing preload by both fluid administration and a head-down position to facilitate return to the right atrium. Any bradycardia should be treated by the delivery of a vagolytic drug. The amount of hypotension that is tolerated depends on the surgical procedure and the preoperative health of the patient to balance oxygen delivery and uptake by the tissues. When the blood pressure cannot be maintained in the correct range during neuraxial anesthesia, this is because of decreased venous return as opposed to the systemic vascular resistance (arteriolar dilatation).[3] Therefore, vasopressor drugs that constrict veins in preference to arterioles are better in treating the hypotension that has resulted. Indirect vasopressors, such as ephedrine, will increase cardiac contractility and cause peripheral vasoconstriction if there are adequate catecholamine stores. These agents offer alpha and beta receptor agonist activity and are potent venoconstrictors. Besides improving the venous return, because of their beta receptor agonist activity, they also increase heart rate. The recommended dose for ephedrine is 5 to 15 mg.

Further treatment consists of further administration of fluid (crystalloid or colloid). Direct vasopressors, such as phenylephrine, cause arteriolar constriction and only minimally increase venous tone with little change or, occasionally, a decrease in the heart rate. The usual dose ranges from 50 to 150 μg (**Box 2**).

PULMONARY SYSTEM

The primary effect of central neural blockade on the lungs depends on the degree of accessory muscle blockade in the thorax. Accessory muscles, like the intercostal muscles, are involved in the inspiration and expiration as well as the anterior abdominal wall musculature. The phrenic nerve is usually spared, except in the rare case where a very high thoracic or cervical epidural has been used for chest or shoulder surgery. Maximum breathing capacity and forced exhalation are decreased in proportion to the amount of accessory muscle blockade that has occurred. The diaphragm can usually maintain the minute volume, tidal volume, and arterial oxygen tension

---

Box 2
Causes of hypotension after neuraxial blockade

Patient Influences

- Baseline pressure less than120 mm Hg
- American Society of Anesthesiologists (ASA) physical status greater than 2
- Hypertension history
- Medications include antihypertensives

Anesthesia Influences

- Block higher than T5
- Additives to the spinal anesthetic, vasoconstrictors, alpha-2
- Combination of general anesthesia and spinal anesthesia[4]

even with a high thoracic blockade. The decrease in ability to actively exhale may be detrimental in a patient with obstructive pulmonary disease. Unfortunately, if this happens in a lightly sedated patient, they may express some degree of anxiety with the feeling of being "unable to breathe" despite the maintenance of ventilation and oxygenation. If possible, with patients with pulmonary disease, it is best to keep the level below T8 to avoid the accessory muscle blockade.

CENTRAL NERVOUS SYSTEM EFFECTS

Cerebral blood flow is autoregulated; therefore, blood flow to the central nervous system should remain constant during central neuraxial blockade unless there is significant hypotension (mean arterial pressure less than about 55 mm Hg in a normal patient).

There is some evidence to support the idea that the neuraxial blockade has some effect on central nervous sedation that is not the direct result of local anesthetic. Both the sevoflurane minimum alveolar concentration dose and the median effective dose of propofol sedation are decreased in the presence of a bupivacaine spinal anesthetic. The amount of sedation produced seems to have a direct correlation to the extent of the spinal blockade.

The effects of central neural blockade on postoperative cognitive dysfunction is harder to differentiate, but may be associated with a decrease in early postoperative cognitive dysfunction. The long-term outcome does not seem to be any different from general anesthesia.

NEUROENDOCRINE EFFECTS

Any trauma and surgical trauma is included in the stress response, which induces the cascade of local and systemic endocrine, metabolic, and immune responses. The stress response can be influenced by the type of surgical anesthesia and the postoperative analgesic regimen. The stress response involves increases in plasma concentration of catabolic hormones such as cortisol, corticotropin, catecholamines, and so forth. The degree of the stress response is directly related to the duration and amount (intensity) of the trauma. It is thought that neuraxial blockade may block the afferent and efferent effects of the stress response and minimize the release of many of the hormonal mediators. Neuraxial anesthesia, in contrast to other types of anesthesia (ie, general, sedation, total intravenous anesthesia) has minimal effect on the stress response.

TEMPERATURE CONSIDERATIONS

Hypothermia is associated with increased myocardial oxygen consumption, increased morbidity, infection, and disruption of the coagulation cascade. Both general anesthesia and central neuraxial blockade seem to impair temperature regulation at the same rate. The major cause of heat loss during spinal and epidural anesthesia is the redistribution of blood flow from the core to the periphery because of the vasodilatation that occurs during central blockade. Because of the blockade of much of the sympathetic system, the usual method of heat control is limited because there is no ability for shivering or vasoconstriction in the area that has the blockade. The central mechanism is also disadvantaged in because the afferent input from the lower body is decreased.

Trying to compare the effects of spinal versus epidural anesthesia seems to lend itself to the belief that the more profound blockade of spinal anesthesia leads to a greater disruption of temperature control in patients who receive spinal anesthesia.

COAGULATION CONCERNS
Preoperative

Much has been written about preoperative considerations for regional anesthesia and most practitioners are guided by the most recent American Society of Regional Anesthesia and Pain Medicine (ASRA) guidelines for regional anesthesia and anticoagulation. Anticoagulation before neuraxial blockade increases the risk of an epidural hematoma and any decision about technique should use some sort of risk-benefit analysis for each individual patient.

Postoperative hypercoagulability is one of the features of the stress response that was discussed and is a major concern for anyone undergoing surgery. Adequate medical decision-making is even being guided by governmental regulations. Immobility and alterations in lower extremity blood flow will contribute to the incidence of thrombotic events. Most postoperative thrombotic and embolic phenomena are begun during the intraoperative care. Neuraxial blockade decreases the risk of thrombotic events during surgery compared with that of general anesthesia. The reasons for this decrease have not been well pinpointed, but are due to some combination of efferent and afferent blockade, effects of the local anesthetic, and alterations of blood flow patterns during spinal and epidural anesthesia (**Box 3**).

The reduction in mean arterial and venous pressures during central neuraxial blockade may be the reason for the documented decrease in blood loss in surgeries for hip replacement and prostatectomy when estimated blood loss has been measured. The postoperative administration of any anticoagulants should be thoroughly discussed with the surgical team so that an appropriate analgesic regimen can be established for a patient if an indwelling catheter will be continued into the postoperative period.

GENITOURINARY EFFECTS

Postoperatively, urinary retention has been a problem for both patients that have received either general or central neuraxial blockade. The bladder is innervated by nerves traveling through the sacral roots. The sympathetic innervation is through the thoracic-lumbar chain and the parasympathetic arises through the sacral level. Blockade can affect urinary sphincter tone and detrusor muscle function. The degree and incidence of bladder disruption is multifactorial depending on age, type of procedure, extent of and choice of blockade, and fluid administration among other variables.

Box 3
Risk factors for thrombosis and emboli postsurgery

Patient Causes

- Preexisting hypercoagulable states
- Secondary hypercoagulable states
- Immobility
- Increased body mass index
- Fracture of pelvis or lower extremity
- Congestive heart failure or cardiac disease
- Birth control pills
- Smoking
- Malignancy

GASTROINTESTINAL EFFECTS

There are mixed opinions on neuraxial blockade, especially those that are continued into the postoperative period and intestinal function. The sympathetic innervation is from the thoracic lumbar chain and the parasympathetic influence is from the vagus stimulation. The blockade and balance of these two competing systems will help determine the outcome.

Because a sympathetic blockade would result in unopposed vagal stimulation, subsequent contracted gut, and possible increase in peristalsis, it was surmised that this increase may be problematic for high surgical anastomosis. However, a retrospective look at leakage after esophagectomy actually showed a slight decrease in the patients who had epidural anesthesia and analgesia. Also, it seems that thoracic epidural analgesia may have a positive effect on bowel function and postoperative ileus compared with that of more traditional opioid analgesia. Every organ system is affected in some way by neuraxial blockade, with more perturbations of organ systems when there is significant blockade of the thoracic system. A thorough understanding of these changes is needed to make the appropriate choice for the patient.

POSTOPERATIVE NEUROLOGIC CONSIDERATIONS

The postoperative neurologic examination has to start preoperatively with a good history and brief examination to evaluate the patient's baseline status. This should include all aspects of his or her medical care if possible. Following the landmark study by Dripps and Vandam,[5] and the resurgence of neuraxial blockade, many studies trying to determine the true incidence of neurologic deficit have been conducted. A multicenter prospective study by Auroy[6] looking at 41,079 spinals and 35,293 epidural anesthetics were performed over a 10-month period using a 24-hour hotline for any complications. This resulted in 31 spinal and 7 epidural events of which there were 10 cardiac arrests and 14 neurologic complications, with more falling into the spinal group. The ASA has reported that approximately 16% of their claims have involved some nerve injury. As with all complications, the reasons are usually multifactorial in nature and make it difficult to identify specific causes.

When there is a neurologic complaint after a spinal or epidural anesthetic, the anesthesiologist is one of the first notified. She or he should be able to provide a comprehensive examination and arrive at a differential diagnosis and should be able to provide direction on what the appropriate course of action should be: further consultation or radiologic imaging.

Frequently, at the author's institution, if we have used the CSE technique, we let our spinal anesthetic regress to the point that we can evaluate neurologic integrity to make sure there has not been any surgical trauma before beginning epidural analgesia. This is to prevent masking a potential problem that would make a differential diagnosis more difficult during the patient's stay.

Neurologic deficits following any neuraxial technique must be included in the differential diagnosis—especially after orthopedic or other lower extremity surgery. The prevalence of nerve injury due to surgery depends both surgical factors and patient-related factors. A meta-analysis of total hip arthroplasties showed an incidence of approximately 1%. This included injuries to the sciatic, femoral, and obturator nerve. Regarding injury to the sciatic nerve, the common peroneal component tends to be more common than injury to the tibial component.

Local anesthetic toxicity can extend from transient neurologic symptoms (TNS) to that of cauda equina syndrome. Cauda equina syndrome can be caused when an exceptionally large dose of a local anesthetic is injected in the subarachnoid space.

Mechanical trauma or direct trauma can happen to the nerve roots or to the conus medullaris ranging from radicular pain to paresthesias or dysesthesias or motor deficits. Reynolds[7] described seven cases of conus injury after a single-shot spinal or CSE using an atraumatic spinal needle. Making sure of correct anatomic landmarks and good technique with respect to the termination of the spinal cord should reduce the incidence of injury.

A thorough neurologic examination postoperatively will include motor and sensory function and evaluation. Diagnostic tests may include an MRI scan. An electromyogram can measure the physiologic function of the motor unit and should help determine where the lesion is located (**Box 4**).

BACK PAIN

Back pain must be taken seriously because this is one of the first complaints of an epidural hematoma; however, most adults experience some degree of back pain during their adult life. Any differential diagnosis for back pain must include preexisting conditions, surgical positioning and technique, anesthesia technique, and drugs that have been used. It may include localized muscular hematoma, ligamentous injury, or local muscle spasm.

Central neuraxial blockade has been associated with local tenderness at the site and is proportional to the size of the needle that has been used. Aching back pain has been described with the use of drugs such as epidural 2-chloroprocaine—containing the preservative ethylenediaminetetraacetic acid—which is believed to be the responsible agent because it binds calcium in the paraspinous tissues.

In a patient who has some preexisting lumbosacral radiculopathy, a well-functioning spinal anesthetic with its associated muscle relaxation may cause additional low back ligamentous strain when placed in the lithotomy position. Perz and colleagues[8] reported a 32% incidence of backache following spinal anesthesia for outpatient surgery. But only 3% of the patients had graded their backache as severe, and about 12% as moderate. Because of this mild nature, spinal anesthesia should not be discouraged for the outpatient population. Once the back pain associated with any major neurologic sequelae has been ruled out, then reassurance, rest, local application of heat and cooling, and analgesics can be applied and is the treatment of choice.

Box 4
Causes of postoperative neurologic deficits

Anesthesia Causes

- Epidural space issues, hematoma, abscess
- Needle trauma, neuropathy
- Local anesthetic toxicity, cauda equina syndrome

Surgery-related causes

- Surgical stretch or compression, retractor injury
- Surgical hematoma causing compression or ischemia
- Positioning injury

Patient-related causes

- Preexisting neuropathies
- Preexisting tumor or lesion, congenital anomaly

Fortunately, backache after central neuraxial blockade is usually transient resolving in 24 to 48 hours with simple conservative therapy.

TRANSIENT NEUROLOGIC SYMPTOMS

As further issues of back pain after spinal anesthesia were investigated, a more formal definition was introduced by Schneider and colleagues[9] in which they reported cases of radicular back pain after hyperbaric spinal anesthesia with lidocaine. All patients were in lithotomy (see previous discussion). All symptoms dissipated within a few days following surgery. A multicenter study was conducted to try to identify the risk factors for TNS. TNS happened more frequently with lidocaine than tetracaine or bupivacaine.[10] The study found that outpatient status, obesity, and lithotomy increased the risk of TNS. These risk factors did not seem to be as evident with tetracaine or bupivacaine (**Box 5**).

MAJOR COMPLICATIONS
Bradycardia and Cardiac Arrest

Bradycardia following central neuraxial blockade may result from normal compensatory mechanisms of arterial and venous baroreceptors coupled with blockade of the preganglionic cardiac accelerators.

A study of over 6000 nonobstetric cases by Lesser and colleagues[11] evaluating the incidence of bradycardia showed an incidence of 9.5% of moderate bradycardia, which was described as heart rate between 40 and 50 beats per minute. Severe bradycardia, with a heart rate less than 40 beats per minute occurred in approximately 0.7%. They were able to identify some risk factors (**Box 6**).

Severe bradycardia in the worst-case scenario may result in cardiac arrest and, as described in the ASA closed claim analysis, the most important factor in resuscitation is the time until the appropriate drug is delivered: atropine, ephedrine, or epinephrine.[12]

ANTERIOR SPINAL ARTERY SYNDROME

The blood supply to the spinal cord is delicate in certain areas. A single midline artery is responsible for supplying much of the blood supply to the anterior portion of the spinal cord. In comparison, the posterior cord is supplied by a pair of longitudinal arteries.

These arteries receive their blood supply from six to seven feeder arteries—the largest is the radicularis magna (artery of Adamkiewicz) to the anterior spinal artery. The artery of Adamkiewicz has individual variation and arises from the aorta between T9 and L2 and supplies most of the conus.

Box 5
Factors that did not increase the risk of TNS after lidocaine spinal anesthesia

- Gender
- Age
- Preexisting back pain
- Needle type or size
- Bevel orientation
- Intrathecal additives (ie, epinephrine, opioids, dextrose)
- Any paresthesia during procedure

Box 6
Risk factors for bradycardia after neuraxial blockade

Moderate bradycardia

- Baseline heart rate, 60
- Male
- Age less than 37 years
- Nonemergent case
- Beta blockade use

Severe bradycardia

- Male
- Baseline heart rate less than 60

The conus is at risk for ischemia when there is a compromise in blood flow by compression, obstruction, or significant hypotension in the face of vascular disease. Anterior spinal artery syndrome affects the motor, pain, and temperature sensation pathways. This may result in a painless loss of movement. Should these signs or symptoms appear, the patient must be immediately evaluated with an MRI and, possibly, an angiogram to discern if there has been a compromise.[13]

SPINAL OR EPIDURAL HEMATOMA OR ABSCESS

The spinal cord is protected by the vertebral bony structures, but this protection can be a detriment when space-occupying lesions within the spinal canal lead to spinal cord or cauda equina compression and ischemia. An epidural abscess or accumulation of blood in the epidural space may cause compression of the cord. Epidural hematomas may occur spontaneously in normal patients or patients with preexisting coagulation disorders, even without any instrumentation. Therefore, careful consideration to all of hemostatic abnormalities must be weighed against the risk and benefits before choosing neuraxial central blockade.

It has been difficult to assess the incidence of hematoma after central neuraxial blockade, but has been estimated to be between 1 in 150,000 and 1 in 200,000.[14] Review of the literature suggests that the risk of hematoma is higher after epidural anesthesia compared with spinal anesthesia. The report of the ASRA consensus Conference on Neuraxial Anesthesia and Anticoagulation evaluated all the available evidence and provides recommendations on the use of various types of medications that can alter coagulation.[15]

Early signs of spinal cord compression include complaints of back pain, progressive sensory or motor blockade, and the onset of bowel or bladder symptoms. If a patient's symptoms do not recede or disappear after resolution of the spinal or epidural, the anesthesiologist should order immediate radiologic imaging and consult with a spine surgeon. Surgical decompression may be warranted and, if this occurs within the first 6 to 12 hours of symptoms, usually the neurologic outcome will be improved.

EPIDURAL OR INTRATHECAL PAIN MANAGEMENT CONSIDERATIONS

The postoperative administration of local anesthetics or opioids or some combination of the two is an excellent way to help control and manage postoperative pain issues for patients. These infusions are especially helpful in thoracic, abdominal pelvic, and most lower extremity orthopedic procedures. There may be some distinct advantages, including early ambulation, preservation of lung function, gastrointestinal benefits, as well as some decrease in thrombosis. A review by Wu and Fleisher[16] concludes that the physiologic and analgesic benefits of postoperative epidural analgesia are affected by its placement at the correct level corresponding to the pain, whether local anesthetic has been added to the infusion, and the length of the time that the infusion is maintained. They noted that, "perioperative epidural anesthesia and analgesia may reduce morbidity and mortality by about 30%."

Opioids are drugs that are most commonly injected into the epidural space or cerebrospinal fluid as a single-shot method for postoperative pain control. There are opioid receptors in the dorsal horn of the spinal cord (Rexed laminae I, II, V).[17] The speed of onset is directly related to the lipid solubility, and dermatomal spread and the duration of action is inversely related to lipid solubility. For example, highly lipid soluble drugs such as fentanyl have a fast onset of action and a short duration, whereas a drug like morphine has a slower onset and longer duration. Because of the short duration of the lipid soluble drugs, morphine is the most commonly used drug by itself for longer postoperative pain management. Because it is hydrophilic, higher concentrations remain in the cerebrospinal fluid as it slowly penetrates the spinal cord (**Table 1**).

A dose of morphine may have the advantage of giving long-term relief to a patient without having multiple doses of parenteral opioids. After intrathecal administration there is very little opioid that can be detected in the bloodstream, which helps minimize some side effects such as sedation. Central opioids do not have an effect on the sympathetic nervous system as do local anesthetics. Therefore, blood pressure and neurologic concerns should not be evident. Ambulation should not be affected. The most serious side effect of central opioids is respiratory depression that happens in dose-dependent fashion. Most serious cases of respiratory depression occur when the patient is receiving other opioids or sedatives after having received intrathecal or epidural opioids. Other side effects include itching nausea, sedation, and urinary retention.

Local anesthetics alone or in combination with opioids are commonly used for postoperative infusions either epidurally or intrathecally. Local anesthetics provide excellent analgesia but, because of their mode of action, can produce both a sympathetic and motor blockade depending on the concentration of the infusion. Dilute local anesthetic solution with or without opioids can provide analgesia with little effect on ambulation. The most commonly used local anesthetics are either bupivacaine in concentrations of .0625% to 25% and ropivacaine in concentrations of 0.1% to 0.2%.

DISCHARGE CRITERIA

The establishment of policies to determine the discharge of a patient to home or to another hospital area after a central blockade is unique to each institution. Each institution must decide what adequate motor blockade regression is and what adequate sensory blockade regression is for the movement of the patient to their next

Table 1 Opioid administration				
Opioid	Oil or Water Partition Coefficient	Dose	Latency (min)	Duration (min)
Morphine	7.9	.05–.25 mg	30–60	480–1440
Fentanyl	8.4	10–50 µg	5–10	30–120
Sufentanil	8.0	2.5–12.5 µg	3–6	60–180

destination. This also applies to the ability of the patient to urinate. The advent of bladder scanning this helped with the individual patients need for urination.

SUMMARY

Spinal and epidural anesthesia and analgesia are indicated for any surgical procedure in which the appropriate sensory level can be accomplished without adverse patient outcomes. When choosing the technique, one must consider the length of the procedure, whether there is a need for postoperative analgesia, and what is most appropriate for the patient's condition. Local anesthetics alone or in combination with opioids are commonly used for postoperative infusions either epidurally or intrathecally.

REFERENCES

1. Lund P. Principles and practice of spinal anesthesia. Springfield (IL): Charles S. Thomas; 1971.
2. Cousins M, Bridenbaugh P. Neural blockade in clinical anesthesia and managemant of pain. 2nd edition. Philadelphia: JB Lippincott; 1992.
3. Ward RJ, Bonica J, Freund FG, et al. Epidural and subarachnoid anesthesia: cardiovascular and respiratory effects. JAMA 1965;191:275–8.
4. Carpenter RL, Caplan RA, Brown DL, et al. Incidence and risk factors for side effects of spinal anesthesia. Anesthesiology 1992;76:906.
5. Dripps RD, Vandam LD. Long-Term follow-up of patient 10,098 spinal anesthetics: failure to discover major neurologic sequelae. JAMA 1954;156:1486–91.
6. Auroy Y, Benhamou D, Bargues L, et al. Major complications of regional anesthesia in France: the SOS regional anesthesia hotlineservice. Anesthesiology 2002;9741:445–52.
7. Reynolds R. Damage to the conus medullaris following spinal anesthesia. Anaesthesia 2001;56:235.
8. Perz RR, Johnson DL, Shinozaki T. Spinal anesthesia for outpatient surgery. Anesth Analg 1988;67:S168.
9. Schneider M, Ettlin T, Kaufman M, et al. Transient neurologic toxicity after hyperbaric subarachnoid anesthesia with 5% lidocaine. Anesth Analg 1993;76:1154–7.
10. Freedman JM, Li DK, Drasner K, et al. Transient neurologic symptoms after spinal anesthesia with lidocaine versus other local anesthetics: a systematic review of randomized controlled trials. Anesth Analg 2005;100:1811–6.
11. Lesser JB, Sanborn KV, Valskys R, et al. Severe bradycardia during spinal and epidural anesthesia recorded by an anesthesia information management system. Anesthesiology 2003;99:859.
12. Caplan RA, Ward RJ, Posner K, et al. Unexpected cardiac arrest during spinal anesthesia. A closed claims analysis of predisposing factors. Anesthesiology 1988;68:5.
13. Hong DK, Lawrence HM. Anterior spinal artery syndrome following total hip arthroplasty under epidural anesthesia. Anaesth Intensive Care 2001;29:62.
14. Vandermeulen EP, Van Aken H, Vermylen J. Anticoagulants and spinal-epidural anesthesia. Anesth Analg 1994;79:1165.
15. Horlocker TT, Wedel DJ, Benzon H, et al. Regional anesthesia in the anticoagulated patient: defining the risks. Reg Anesth Pain Med 2003;28:172.
16. Wu CL, Fleisher LA. Outcomes research in regional anesthesia. Anesth Analg 2000;91:1232.
17. Cousins MJ, Mather LE. Intrathecal and epidural administration of opioids. Anesthesiology 1984;61:276.

Perioperative Glycemic Control

Nicholas Russo, MD[a,b,*]

KEYWORDS

- Glycemic control • Blood glucose • Surgery • Diabetes mellitus

KEY POINTS

- Perioperative hyperglycemia has potential significant adverse consequences of increased mortality and morbidity including surgical site infection, renal insufficiency and anemia requiring transfusion.
- Both diabetic and non-diabetic patients are affected adversely by perioperative hyperglycemia. However, these two subgroups do not necessarily benefit equally from perioperative glycemic control.
- The ideal target glucose range as well as the appropriate patient population(s) for whom glycemic control offers the most benefit have yet to be fully elucidated. However, there are clear potential adverse consequences of tight control such as hypoglycemia.

INTRODUCTION

Blood glucose (BG) levels are tightly regulated within a narrow range (60–90 mg/dL), and long-term deviation from this norm has well-defined and potentially severe adverse consequences manifested as the clinical complications of diabetes mellitus.[1] Those individuals with fasting BG (FBG) levels that lie outside this range are categorized into 2 classes as defined by the American College of Endocrinology and the American Diabetes Association. These are a prediabetic state (FBG 100–125 mg/dL) and true diabetes mellitus (FBG $\geq$126).[2] It is estimated that as many as 13% of the United States population fit diabetic criteria, but 40% of these individuals are unaware that they carry such a diagnosis.[3] In addition, 26% of the population meets prediabetic criteria, of whom 60% to 70% progress to fulminant diabetes.[4]

The prevalence of glycemic dysregulation, and consequently the number of individuals with the myriad chronic complications of diabetes, is significant. Diabetic patients experience more frequent perioperative complications.[5,6] However, perioperative acute hyperglycemia in both diabetics and nondiabetics is an independent predictor of morbidity and mortality.[7–9] Increased BG levels can lead to several adverse results such as osmotic diuresis, fluid and electrolyte imbalances, and impaired wound healing and immune function. In addition, reducing hyperglycemia in diabetics reduces

[a] Intensive Care Unit, Medina General Hospital, 1000 E. Washington St, Medina, OH 44256, USA;
[b] Anesthesia Critical Care Institute, Cleveland Clinic Foundation, 9500 Euclid Ave, Cleveland, OH 44195, USA
* Anesthesia Critical Care Institute, Cleveland Clinic Foundation, Cleveland, OH.
E-mail address: russon@ccf.org

Anesthesiology Clin 30 (2012) 445–466
http://dx.doi.org/10.1016/j.anclin.2012.07.007
1932-2275/12/$ – see front matter © 2012 Elsevier Inc. All rights reserved.
anesthesiology.theclinics.com

microvascular and macrovascular complications,[10-16] and perioperative glycemic control in both groups improves rates of nosocomial and wound infections.[17-26]

HISTORICAL SYNOPSIS

Glycemic control was originally investigated in diabetic patients because of the observation that this group was particularly susceptible to certain infections and infectious complications[14,21] (eg, postoperative wound infections). This vulnerability was shown to be the result of compromised immunity; in particular, impaired polymorphonuclear leukocyte function, chemotaxis, and phagocytosis.[21-26]

When comparing operative mortality and complications (eg, wound infection, myocardial infarction, dysrhythmias, and respiratory failure) between diabetic and nondiabetic patients undergoing coronary artery bypass grafting (CABG), investigators in 1991 found that the 2 groups had no mortality difference; however, the diabetics experienced significantly increased morbidity most prominently with regard to wound infections.[11] In a before-and-after chart review, the rate of deep sternal wound infections in diabetic patients undergoing CABG was examined following the implementation of a strict glycemic control protocol. With a glucose target of 200 mg/dL, researchers found reduced infection rates as well as reduced morbidity and associated cost after initiation of the protocol.[15]

Two more studies done in 1998 and 1999 also showed the potential relationship between perioperative glycemic control and postoperative infection rates. The data in one showed that diabetic patients with a BG level greater than 220 mg/dL on postoperative day 1 had more than a 2.5-fold increased risk of nosocomial infections.[13] In the other, data revealed that diabetic patients undergoing CABG with a postoperative glucose greater than 200 mg/dL had increased infection rates.[14] These early results investigating the relationship between perioperative hyperglycemia, glycemic control, and infection and mortality in surgical and critically ill patients are shown in **Table 1**.

The historical connection between diabetics who experience perioperative hyperglycemia and adverse perioperative outcomes is strong.[27,28] However, several studies have shown a link between perioperative hyperglycemia (BG >200 mg/dL) and negative outcomes regardless of diabetic status.[29-31] Moreover, approximately 10% to 15% of those patients without diabetes experience perioperative hyperglycemia. Two early retrospective analyses found evidence that hyperglycemia (BG >200 mg/dL) on the day of surgery was associated with increased mortality and morbidity (eg, stroke and myocardial infarction) during surgery.[29,32]

The prior beliefs that hyperglycemia was simply a response to physiologic stressors and that higher glucose levels were necessary to fuel glucose dependent organs slowly shifted to one of possible cause and effect. As a result of this apparent relationship, intensive perioperative glucose control has been proposed and studied extensively because of its potential to mitigate perioperative complications.

In 2001, Van den Berghe and colleagues[33] published a randomized controlled trial (RCT) with more than 1500 patients in a surgical intensive care unit (ICU) setting who received intensive glycemic control and experienced a 34% reduction in hospital mortality when compared with traditional therapy. In addition, the investigators noted reduced perioperative complications including blood stream infections, acute renal failure, red blood cell transfusions, critical illness polyneuropathy, and reduced duration of ventilatory support.[33] Subsequently, additional investigators have found a reduction in infectious complications with improved survival attributable to intensive glucose control in the cardiac surgical population[15,34-36] along with improved outcomes in the settings of acute neurologic injury and acute myocardial infarction.

Table 1
Infection rate and mortality in clinical trials of hyperglycemia and infection in surgical and critically ill patients

Trial Design (Year)	Study Type	Patient Population	Primary End Point	Results
Nonrandomized, retrospective (1991)[11]	Observational	Diabetic and nondiabetic patients undergoing CABG (n = 711, 146 diabetic vs 565 nondiabetic)	Mortality within 30 d of surgery or during same hospitalization	No difference in mortality. Higher morbidity and wound infection rate in diabetic vs nondiabetic patients
Prospective, nonrandomized, cohort (1998)[13]	Observational	Diabetic patients undergoing elective surgery (n = 93)	Relationship between glucose control and development of postoperative nosocomial infections (bacteremia, UTI, pneumonia, surgical wound infection, intra-abdominal abscess, Clostridium difficile colitis)	Higher infection rate (except for UTI) in patients with BGL >220 mg/dL vs BGL <220 mg/dL on postoperative day 1
Nonconcurrent, prospective, cohort, blinded (1999)[14]	Observational	Diabetic patients undergoing CABG (n = 411)	Relationship between perioperative glycemic control and development of postoperative infectious complications (eg, pneumonia, UTI, wound infection) on day 2 or ≥36 h after surgery	Higher overall infection rate and infectious complications corresponding with higher BGL
Nonrandomized, retrospective, case-control (2000)[16]	Observational	Diabetic and nondiabetic patients undergoing CABG (n = 120. 30 case patients with deep sternal site infection, 90 control patients)	Deep sternal site infection rate before and during study period	Lower deep sternal site infection rate before vs during study period
Nonrandomized, retrospective, case-control (2000)[17]	Observational	Diabetic and nondiabetic patients undergoing radial artery graft for revascularization during CABG (n = 127, 35 case patients, 92 control patients)	Development of radial artery harvest site infection after CABG during heightened and routine postdischarge surveillance	Higher rate of radial artery harvest site infection during heightened vs routine surveillance

(continued on next page)

Table 1
(continued)

Trial Design (Year)	Study Type	Patient Population	Primary End Point	Results
Prospective, cohort, blinded, case-control (2001)[18]	Observational	Patients with known DM, unknown DM, and nondiabetic patients with hyperglycemia undergoing CABG or cardiac valve procedure (n = 1044, 300 with known DM, 700 with unknown DM, 44 DM status not mentioned; 74 infected, 970 control)	Development of surgical site infection as related to BGL control (BGL and hemoglobin A_{1c})	Frequency of surgical site infections directly and significantly correlated with degree of hyperglycemia during postoperative period. Higher surgical site infection rate in patients with known DM vs patients with unknown DM. Higher surgical site infection rate in patients with known and unknown DM and nondiabetic patients
Retrospective, cohort (2002)[85]	Observational	Diabetic and nondiabetic patients undergoing CABG (n = 1090, 400 diabetic, 690 nondiabetic patients)	Postoperative infectious complications (deep and superficial sternal wound infection, donor site infection, UTI, lung infection) as related to perioperative and postoperative glycemic control	Diabetic: higher perioperative BGL correlated with higher deep sternal wound infection rate. Higher postoperative infection rate (deep sternal wound infection, donor site infection, UTI) in diabetic vs nondiabetic patients. Higher early mortality in diabetic vs nondiabetic patients
Historical cohort (2003)[19]	Observational	Diabetic and nondiabetic patients undergoing CABG (n = 1574, 545 diabetic, 1029 nondiabetic patients)	30-d mortality, 30-d infections (harvest site, sepsis, pneumonia, UTI, deep sternal wound infection), resource use as related to perioperative hyperglycemia	Higher overall infection rate in diabetic vs nondiabetics patients. Higher mortality in patients who developed infection in both groups
Prospective, 1 center (2003)[38]	Observational	Diabetic and nondiabetic patients admitted to cardiothoracic, cardiorespiratory surgery, and medicine ICU (n = 523)	ICU mortality	In all glucose bands, increased insulin administration corresponded with significantly increased risk of ICU death

Retrospective, longitudinal, 1 center (2003)[37]	Observational	Diabetic and nondiabetic patients admitted to general medical, surgical, and coronary ICU (n = 1826)	Hospital mortality	Higher BGL, corresponded with higher hospital mortality
Nonrandomized, retrospective (1997)[12]	Interventional: insulin protocol, BGL goal <200 mg/dL	Diabetic and nondiabetic patients undergoing cardiac surgery (n = 8910, 1585 diabetic, 7325 nondiabetic patients)	Deep sternal wound infection rate before and after diabetic protocol	Diabetic: higher deep sternal wound infection rate before vs after protocol. Nondiabetic: higher deep sternal wound infection rate before vs after protocol
Nonrandomized, prospective (1999)[15]	Interventional: insulin protocol, BGL goal 150–200 mg/dL	Diabetic patients undergoing open heart surgery (n = 2467, 968 control, 1499 continuous insulin infusion)	Infection (deep and superficial sternal wound infection, donor site infection) rate as related to postoperative BGL before and after protocol	Higher deep sternal wound infection rate in control vs continuous insulin infusion group
Prospective, randomized, controlled (2001)[32]	Interventional: insulin protocol, intensive group BGL goal 80–110 mg/dL; conventional group BGL goal 180–200 mg/dL	Diabetic and nondiabetic surgical patients in ICUs (n = 1548, 765 intensive insulin, 783 conventional insulin)	Death from any cause during ICU stay	Lower overall ICU mortality, lower mortality in patients in ICU >5 d, lower overall in-hospital mortality, lower in-hospital mortality in patients in ICU >5 d, lower frequency of septicemia, prolonged antibiotics, and bacteremia in intensive vs conventional group
Nonrandomized, historical control (2004)[39]	Interventional: insulin protocol, BGL goal <140 mg/dL	Diabetic and nondiabetic surgical and medical patients in ICUs (n = 1600, 800 historical control, 800 treatment group)	In-hospital mortality before and after protocol	Lower hospital mortality after protocol implementation. Infection rate similar before and after protocol

Abbreviations: BGL, blood glucose level; DM, diabetes mellitus; ICU, intensive care unit; UTI, urinary tract infection.

In 2003, a study completed by Van den Berghe and colleagues[36] examined the relative contributions of insulin dosage versus level of hyperglycemia to the proposed outcome benefits seen 2 years earlier. Their results showed that it was the control of hyperglycemia rather than the dose of insulin that was associated with the improvements in mortality, polyneuropathy, and anemia. However, the reduction in acute renal failure did not follow this relationship[37] and the mechanism for improvement in this parameter remains unclear. Also in 2003, a 6-month, prospective, observational study was reported. This trial examined the extent to which insulin administration and glucose control determined patient outcome.[38] The investigators found a positive and significant correlation between insulin dosage and mortality, suggesting that glycemic control rather than insulin administration offered survival benefit. In addition, they noted that mortality was increased at a glucose level of more than 145 mg/dL to 180 mg/dL.[38]

In that same year, Krinsley[39] examined a heterogeneous critical care population. First, retrospectively, he observed that even modest increases in mean glucose concentrations correlated with increased mortality. Then, using a historical control group, they reviewed the effect of a glycemic control protocol, revealing decreased hospital mortality, acute renal failure, and ICU length of stay.[40] However, this failed to show improvement in the incidence of infection.

Several studies have investigated an antiinflammatory role for insulin administration through the modulation of C-reactive protein[41] or through suppression of proinflammatory cytokine and superoxide radical production.[37,42,43]

Although these data were promising and the concept generated enthusiastic resource allocation to intensive glycemic control protocol creation and implementation, potential adverse consequences of such tight regulation and the uncertainty surrounding optimal glucose targets have recently been encountered.[44–46]

In 2006, Van den Berghe and colleagues[45,46] examined intensive glycemic control in a medical ICU setting. Medical critical care patients did not have the same benefits as the surgical critical care population. In addition, and perhaps more importantly, 2 separate studies had to be stopped early by their respective data safety boards because of frequent severe hypoglycemia (BG ≤40 mg/dL). Furthermore, in 2007, Gandhi and colleagues[46] found that intraoperative intensive glycemic control during cardiac surgery may increase the incidence of death and stroke.

Thus, given the variability in outcomes and potential for deleterious side effects and complications, the aforementioned mobilization of resources toward intensive glycemic control protocols may have been premature. Thus, this article reviews the pathophysiology and potential detrimental effects of acute perioperative hyperglycemia and discusses the available evidence for preoperative, intraoperative, and critical care intensive glycemic control.

PATHOPHYSIOLOGY OF PERIOPERATIVE HYPERGLYCEMIA

Under stress conditions such as surgery, trauma, sepsis, and critical illness, hyperglycemia becomes prevalent, partly because of significant perturbations in glucose metabolism. Increased sympathetic nervous system activity coupled with enhanced release of counterregulatory hormones both contribute to a hyperglycemic state. This effect is modulated through the processes of gluconeogenesis and glycogenolysis in various organs such as skeletal muscle and the liver. Inflammatory cytokines inhibit insulin release and thus contribute to relative insulin resistance. These physiologic alterations drive stress-induced hyperglycemia.[22,48–51]

Insulin resistance has been shown to rapidly develop following noncardiac operations of intermediate risk and duration.[52] Thorell and colleagues[53] showed that insulin resistance in patients undergoing cholecystectomy became most prominent on post-operative day 1 and lasted for between 9 and 21 days (insulin sensitivity was 50% of baseline). The degree of insulin resistance and the perioperative hyperglycemic response has been shown to be directly related to the degree of surgical trauma.[54,55]

The operative approach as well as a laparoscopic versus open technique contribute to varying degrees of hyperglycemia.[56,57] In addition, thoracic and abdominal procedures have been shown to drive a more robust and prolonged hyperglycemic state than lower risk peripheral or diagnostic procedures.[54] This apparent variation based on surgical site may be explained by differing inflammatory and stress responses; for example, cardiac surgery with cardiopulmonary bypass under deep hypothermic arrest is an extreme scenario with profound inflammatory and stress responses that both reduce insulin secretion and increase insulin resistance.[58]

Perioperative hyperglycemia may also be the result of underlying patient factors such as diabetes, obesity, and acute pancreatitis. It may also be iatrogenic from the administration of catecholamines, parenteral nutrition, or corticosteroids. **Fig. 1** provides a summary of the various pathophysiologic causes of perioperative hyperglycemia.

GLYCEMIC CONTROL IN THE CRITICALLY ILL

In a potentially landmark event in 2001, Van den Berghe and colleagues[33] compared intensive glycemic control (BG of 80–110 mg/dL) with conventional therapy (BG target of 180–200 mg/dL) in more than 1500 surgical patients in ICUs receiving mechanical ventilation. Their data showed a 34% reduction in in-hospital mortality as well as a significant reduction in several morbidity parameters. The parameters included a reduced incidence of bloodstream infection, acute renal failure requiring renal replacement therapy, blood transfusion, and critical illness polyneuropathy. In addition, the treatment group experienced shorter duration of mechanical ventilation as well as ICU length of stay (LOS). Furthermore, when a subsequent before-and-after historical case-control study showed a 29% reduction in hospital mortality[40] with similarly improved morbidity parameters, albeit with a less restrictive BG target (BG 80–140 mg/dL), this offered credence to the reproducibility of the Van den Berghe and colleagues[33] data.

In the 2001 study, the adverse consequence of intensive glycemic control were primarily hypoglycemia (BG ≤40 mg/dL, 5.1% in the treatment group vs 0.8% in the control). Further, additional challenges to the ability to generalize the data have been posed. First, it was performed at a single center and was not blinded. Second, most patients (63%) had had cardiac surgery; and, third, the nurse/patient ratio was 1:1, which is higher than in most ICUs. In addition, although both the control and treatment groups were subjected to high-dextrose infusions and parenteral nutrition on the day of surgery and first postoperative day, there was the concern that the outcome differences were enhanced because of the control group receiving an unconventional treatment. It has been proposed that the disproportionate allocation of resources and personnel prevented a higher incidence of hypoglycemia as well as more significant adverse consequences.[58,59]

After this, Van den Berghe and colleagues[44] undertook another study in 2006 that examined intensive glycemic control (BG 80–110 mg/dL) against conventional therapy (BG 180–200 mg/dL) in 1200 medical patients in ICUs. The results of this study revealed a reduction in morbidity parameters similar to the 2001 endeavor[33] (ie, reduced ICU LOS, renal failure, and ventilator days), but an overall mortality reduction could not be shown as before. However, after further subgroup analysis, a mortality benefit was afforded to those patients with an ICU LOS of 3 days or greater (53%

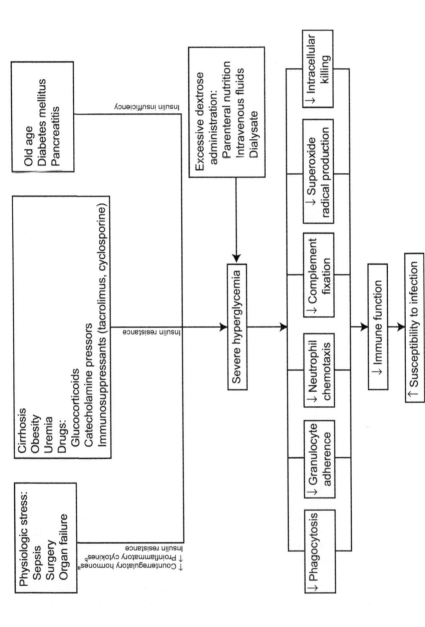

Fig. 1. Causes of hyperglycemia and effects of hyperglycemia on increased susceptibility to infection in the critically ill patient. [a] Counterregulatory hormones are glucagon, catecholamines, cortisol, and growth hormone, [b] Proinflammatory cytokines are tumor necrosis factor, interleukin (IL)-1 and IL-6. (*From* Butler SO, Btaiche IF, Alaniz C. Relationship between hyperglycemia and infection in critically ill patients. Pharmacotherapy 2005;25(7): 963–76; with permission.)

vs 45%), but those with an ICU LOS of less than 3 days had a trend toward increased mortality and a priori classification of patients was not possible.

The medical ICU investigation also realized increased incidence of hypoglycemia in the intensive glycemic control group (18.7% vs 3.1% in control) but, possibly most importantly in this study, a multivariate analysis revealed hypoglycemia as an independent predictor of mortality. Although the mechanism by which this occurred was unable to be identified, this study was the first to show the possible harm of intensive glycemic control.

Subsequent studies have also revealed hypoglycemia to be an independent predictor of mortality; in addition, these trials have identified risk factors other than intensive glycemic control that are associated with hypoglycemia. One such study identified continuous renal replacement therapy, diabetes, sepsis, and vasopressor support as independent predictors of hypoglycemia.[60] Krinsley and colleagues[61] found similar predictors of hypoglycemia but, through a multivariate analysis of their study data, the connection between hypoglycemia and mortality was reasserted.

Another study evaluating intensive glycemic control was halted early as a result of increased incidence of hypoglycemia and other complications. A European study of intensive glycemic control in a mixed medical-surgical ICU population stopped early as a result of increased hypoglycemia in the treatment group. This study initially found that hypoglycemia was associated with increased mortality, a result that was revised after further analysis to simply no mortality benefit from intensive control.[62]

In addition, a meta-analysis of 29 randomized trials of intensive glycemic control versus conventional therapy failed to show an in-hospital mortality benefit regardless of glucose goal or patient population.[63] However, it did identify a reduced incidence of sepsis in surgical patients in ICUs, albeit with a 5-fold worse rate of hypoglycemia.

Table 2 provides a summary of intensive glycemic control data in the ICU population.

INTRAOPERATIVE INTENSIVE GLYCEMIC CONTROL

Although intensive glycemic management has been extensively evaluated across the spectrum of ICU patient populations, the data for a similar style of glycemic control in the intraoperative setting are lacking and exist exclusively in the cardiac surgical population. In patients having cardiac surgery, a mortality benefit was initially recognized in patients who had had myocardial infarction and stroke who received a glucose-insulin-potassium mixture.[64,65] However, because of how these early investigations were designed (ie, with the rationale of studying the cardioprotective effects of this mixture based on its metabolic and biochemical cellular results), glycemic control was not an a priori end point[65–67] and thus the investigators were unable to establish a link between hyperglycemia and morbidity and mortality.

In a before-and-after study, Furnary and colleagues[68] examined data from a larger project (The Portland Diabetic Project, a prospective, nonrandomized interventional study) and compared intraoperative intensive glycemic control with standard subcutaneous insulin in historical control diabetic patients undergoing CABG. Their results showed a 57% reduction in mortality.[69] However, because of the nonrandomized nature of the study as well as protocol changes during the study period (BG targets initially were <200 mg/dL, then later changed to 100–150 mg/dL), the validity of these results has been questioned.

Another before-and-after study examined patients undergoing CABG and subjected to intensive glycemic control both during and after surgery.[70] This investigation found a 72% mortality benefit. Several additional studies have related poor intraoperative glycemic control in patients undergoing CABG to increased mortality and

Table 2
Studies of intensive insulin therapy in the critically ill

Study	Design	Patient Population	Primary End Point	Major Findings
Van den Berghe, et al,[32] 2001	Single-center RCT. partially blinded of IIT (target BG, 80–110 mg/dL) vs conventional treatment (insulin infusion if BG >215 mg/dL, with target BG 180–200)	1548 surgical patients in ICUs receiving mechanical ventilation	Death from any cause during intensive care	IIT reduced mortality in the ICU from 8.0% to 4.6% ($P < .04$), in-hospital mortality by 34%, bloodstream infections by 46%, ARF requiring dialysis or hemofiltration by 41%, red-cell transfusions by 50%, and polyneuropathy by 44%
Van den Berghe et al,[43] 2006	Single-center RCT of IIT (target BG, 80–110 mg/dL) vs conventional treatment (insulin infusion if BG >215 mg/dL; with target BG 180–200 mg/dL)	1200 patients admitted to medical ICU thought to need intensive care for at least 3 d	Death from any cause in the hospital	No reduction in in-hospital mortality in intention-to-treat analysis. Among patients who stayed in ICU for >3 d, there was a decrease in mortality from 52.5% to 43% ($P = .009$) in the treatment group; among those staying <3 d, treatment group mortality was greater
Van den Berghe et al,[86] 2006	Pooled dataset analysis of 2 RCTs comparing IIT (target BG 80–110 mg/dL) with conventional treatment (insulin infusion if BG >215 mg/dL; target BG 180–200 mg/dL)	Pooled data of 2748 medical and surgical patients in ICUs from 2 RCTs	Goals to investigate harm in brief treatment in mixed population, identify subgroups who may not benefit from IIT, to determine optimal target BG, and to study hypoglycemia	IIT decreased mortality in intention-to-treat group (20.4% vs 23.6%; $P = .04$); short stayers had no difference in mortality; mortality was higher with BG >150 mg/dL and lower with BG <110 mg/dL compared with BG 110–150 mg/dL; patients with diabetes showed no benefit; hypoglycemia was more likely with target BG <110 mg/dL and was not associated with morbidity

Krinsley[39] 2004	Before-after study of intensive glucose management protocol (target BG <140 mg/dL maintained with SC insulin unless BG >200 mg/dL on 2 successive fingersticks	1600 patients in university-affiliated community hospital mixed medical/surgical ICU	Hospital mortality	After implementation of the protocol, hospital mortality decreased 29.3% ($P = .002$), LOS in ICU decreased 10.8% ($P = .01$), incidence of new renal insufficiency decreased 18.7% ($P = .04$), and red-cell transfusions decreased 18.7% ($P = .04$); there was no significant change in the incidence of hypoglycemia
Finney et al,[37] 2003	Single-center, prospective observational study of effects of glycemic control and insulin administration	531 patients admitted to mixed medical/surgical ICU	ICU mortality	Increased administration of insulin was associated with increased ICU mortality (OR 1.02; $P<.001$) in normoglycemic patients (BG 111–144 mg/dL)
Krinsley and Grover,[60] 2007	Retrospective database review and case-control analysis of risk factors for severe hypoglycemia (BG <40 mg/dL) before and after implementation of tight glycemic control protocol (target BG 80–140 mg/dL, then 80–125 mg/dL)	102 patients in medical/surgical ICU with severe hypoglycemia from a series of 5365 patients	N/A	Treatment in tight glycemic control period is an independent risk factor for severe hypoglycemia, and severe hypoglycemia is an independent predictor of mortality (OR 2.28; $P = .0008$)
Toft et al,[87] 2006	Prospective before-after study of IIT (target BG 80–110 mg/dL) vs conventional therapy (target BG <216 mg/dL)	271 noncardiac patients in ICUs	ICU mortality	Study was underpowered, but it showed a trend toward reduced mortality and decreased incidence of infection. Hypoglycemia was significantly more common in the IIT group (14% vs 4%)

(continued on next page)

Table 2
(continued)

Study	Design	Patient Population	Primary End Point	Major Findings
Ingels et al,[88] 2006	Preplanned subanalysis of patients having cardiac surgery from first Leuven study	970 patients admitted to the ICU after cardiac surgery	4-year all-cause mortality and number of posthospital discharge deaths	Mortality at 4 y was similar among groups; among patients staying in ICU at least 3 d, mortality at 4 y was lower for IIT group (23% vs 36%); posthospital discharge deaths were similar; increased survival among long stayers was associated with decreased perceived quality of life
Brunkhorst et al,[44] 2008	Multicenter 2 × 2 factorial trial, randomly assigning patients to IIT or conventional therapy and either 10% pentastarch or modified Ringer lactate	Analysis of patients with severe sepsis or septic shock admitted to multidisciplinary ICUs at 18 hospitals: n = 488 for insulin arm, n = 537 for fluid arm	Death at 28 d and mean score for organ failure	Stopped early for safety reasons; no difference in rate of death or mean score for organ failure at 28 d; rate of severe hypoglycemia (BG <40 mg/dL) was higher in treatment group (17% vs 4.1%; $P<.001$), as was rate of serious adverse events (10.9% vs 5.2%, $P = .01$)
Glucontrol[a] Trial,[89]	Single-blinded, multicenter, RCT of IIT (target BG 80–110 mg/dL) vs conventional therapy (target BG 140–180 mg/dL)	Goal to enroll 3500 patients; stopped after 1101 medical/surgical patients in ICUs at 21 hospitals completed the study	ICU mortality	Stopped early for safety reasons and a high rate of protocol violations; incidence of severe hypoglycemia increased in treatment arm (8.6% vs 2.4%; $P<.001$); no difference in all-cause mortality or LOS
Lazar et al,[70] 2004	Prospective randomized trial of intraoperative glucose-insulin-potassium (target BG 125–200) or standard therapy (BG <250)	141 diabetic patients undergoing CABG	Perioperative outcomes	Patients receiving glucose-insulin-potassium have a lower incidence of A-Fib, shorter postoperative LOS, few recurrent wound infections, and improved survival at 2 y

Study	Description	Patients	Outcome	Results
Furnary et al,[68] 2003	Before-after study of intraoperative subcutaneous insulin vs continuous insulin infusion (target BG range changed during study period: 150–200 → 125–175 → 100–150 mg/dL)	3554 diabetic patients undergoing CABG	In-hospital mortality	Continuous insulin infusion was independently predictive against death (OR 0.34; $P = .001$), and observed mortality was less than expected by the Society of Thoracic Surgeons' 1996 multivariable risk model (observed/expected = 0.63; $P<.001$)
Ouattara et al,[33] 2005	Prospective trial of intraoperative intravenous insulin therapy (initiated for BG ≥180 mg/dL)	200 consecutive diabetic patients undergoing on-pump CABG	Severe CV, respiratory, infectious, neurologic, and renal in-hospital morbidity	Adjusted OR for severe postoperative morbidity in patients with poor intraoperative glycemic control (defined as 4 consecutive BG >200 mg/dL) was 7.2 (95% CI 2.7–19.0)
Gandhi et al,[34] 2005	Retrospective observational study with independent variable mean intraoperative BG	409 consecutive patients having cardiac surgery	Composite of death and infectious, neurologic, renal, cardiac, and pulmonary complications developing within 30 d of surgery	Intraoperative hyperglycemia is an independent risk factor for complications and death after cardiac surgery (adjusted OR for composite outcome, 1.34 for each 20-mg/dL increase in mean intraoperative BG; 95% CI, 1.10–1.62)

(continued on next page)

Table 2
(continued)

Study	Design	Patient Population	Primary End Point	Major Findings
Doenst et al,[35] 2005	Retrospective observational study	1579 diabetic and 4701 nondiabetic patients undergoing on-pump cardiac surgery	In-hospital mortality	Increased glucose is an independent predictor of mortality in diabetic (OR 1.20 per 1-mmol increase in BG; $P = .0005$) and nondiabetic (OR = 1.12; $P<.0001$) patients
Gandhi et al,[46] 2007	Open-label, single-center RCT with blinded end point assessment; continuous insulin infusion to keep intraoperative BG 80–100 mg/dL vs conventional treatment (BG <200 mg/dL)	400 patients undergoing on-pump cardiac surgery	Composite of death, sternal infections, prolonged ventilation, cardiac arrhythmias, stroke, and renal failure within 30 d after surgery	No difference in number of events between groups; intensive insulin group trended toward more deaths (4 vs 0; $P = .061$) and had higher incidence of stroke (8 vs 1; $P = .020$)

Abbreviations: A-Fib, atrial fibrillation; ARF, acute renal failure; CI, confidence interval; CV, cardiovascular; IIT, intensive insulin therapy; OR, odds ratio; SC, subcutaneous.

[a] Glucontrol Study: comparing the effects of 2 glucose control regimens by insulin in patients in ICUs. Available at: http://clinicaltrials.gov/ct/gui/show/NCT00107601. Accessed July 18, 2008.

severely increased in-hospital morbidity. These studies suggest that glycemic control initiated in the intraoperative period may provide a survival advantage as well as decreased LOS and reduced wound infection rates.[12,35,36] However, the results are less robust, because 1 study was not blinded and had potential undertreatment of the standard therapy group,[12] and the others were retrospective in nature.[35,36]

In contrast, Gandhi and colleagues[47] published a prospective RCT investigating intensive glycemic control (BG 80–110 mg/dL) versus standard therapeutic range (BG <200 mg/dL) in both diabetic and nondiabetic patients undergoing CABG in which there was no difference in perioperative morbidity or mortality. Their data showed a trend toward increased mortality and a higher incidence of stroke in the intensive glycemic control group.

Only retrospective and observational data exist supporting the hypothesis that intraoperative intensive glycemic control improves perioperative outcomes. Prospective data are scant and show no mortality benefit and a trend toward increasing perioperative morbidity.[47] A more robust prospective data set may answer whether intensive glycemic control applied during surgery improves perioperative outcomes.

POSTOPERATIVE INTENSIVE GLYCEMIC CONTROL

Glycemic control in the postoperative period has been shown to reduce wound infections and postoperative hyperglycemia has been associated with poor outcomes. Hyperglycemia as a result of neuroendocrine physiology and the stress response to surgical procedures is most notable in the postoperative period.

A before-and-after study of more than 1500 diabetic patients undergoing cardiac surgery showed a lower incidence of deep wound infection after initiation of an insulin protocol with a target BG of less than 200 mg/dL.[71] Furnary and colleagues,[15] in a prospective investigation, showed a 66% reduction in sternal wound infection, whereas a retrospective investigation supported hyperglycemia as an independent predictor of postoperative infection in diabetic patients undergoing cardiac surgery.[14]

Although investigations of intensive glycemic control outside the perioperative and critical care populations are sparse, 1 prospective study in 834 patients undergoing surgical clipping of cerebral aneurysm after subarachnoid hemorrhage found a reduced infection rate in the intensive glycemic control group (BG 80–120 mg/dL) compared with conventional therapy (BG 80–220 mg/dL).[72] However, the investigators found no improvement in mortality or other morbidity parameters (eg, vasospasm).

As discussed earlier, the strongest data set in favor of intensive postoperative glycemic control (and also in the critical care setting) is the prospective study by Van den Berghe and colleagues.[73] However, the results of this study have been challenged because caregivers were not blinded to therapy, patients received large amounts of exogenous glucose and enteral/parenteral nutrition, and the control group experienced unusually high mortality based on disease severity.

Given the results of Van den Berghe and colleagues[73] together with the myriad retrospective cardiac surgical data supporting the association between hyperglycemia and poor perioperative outcomes, resources were aggressively allocated to the development and implementation of intensive glycemic control protocols; intensive glycemic control was thought to be beneficial in almost all critically ill postsurgical patients.

As stated previously, Van den Berghe and colleagues[45,46] published a study in 2006 evaluating the impact of intensive glycemic control in the medical ICU population.[44] The trial did not show the anticipated mortality benefit seen previously in surgical critical care patients, but provided data on hypoglycemia as an independent predictor of mortality. In addition, the Normoglycemia in Intensive Care Evaluation and Survival

Using Glucose Algorithm Regulation (NICE-SUGAR)[74] study evaluated intensive glycemic control (BG 81–108 mg/dL) versus conventional therapy (BG 144–180 mg/dL) in more than 6000 mixed medical/surgical critical care patients. The study was unable to show a significant difference between the groups in the categories of 90-day mortality, LOS (both in hospital and ICU), and the need for renal replacement therapy. The study found increased mortality in the intensive glycemic control group (27.5% vs 24.9%, odds ratio [OR] = 1.14, 95% confidence interval [CI] 1.02–1.28) and no difference in the surgical population on subgroup analysis. In addition, even though the relationship between hypoglycemia and mortality has yet to be disclosed for this trial, it did find an incidence of hypoglycemia that was 13 times higher in the treatment group.

The NICE-SUGAR study results coupled with data from a recent meta-analysis[75] and the association between hypoglycemia and mortality found in the second trial by Van den Berghe and colleagues[45,46] cast doubt on the practice of intensive glycemic control in the critical care population. A meta-analysis including the NICE-SUGAR data failed to show a mortality benefit to intensive glycemic control but reiterated a 6-fold increased incidence in hypoglycemia.

HYPOGLYCEMIA

Low BG levels are known to have a deleterious effect on organ function and, in particular, the function of the brain. However, during the perioperative period and critical illness, hypoglycemia may go unrecognized, resulting in irreversible brain injury and mortality.[76,77] Hypoglycemia normally results in a compensatory response that mimics the clinical picture frequently seen in patients in the early postoperative period or those experiencing critical illness. This response may alternatively be blunted because of pharmacologic intervention such as with sedatives and analgesics. In addition, in the setting of ischemia, as may occur with shock states, the brain resorts to production and use of lactate from glucose as its energy source. If glucose levels are greatly and abruptly lowered, as may be the case with intensive glycemic control, ischemic brain injury may be worsened.

TARGET SERUM GLUCOSE LEVELS

With the data presented earlier, it is more and more evident that the aggressive BG target of less than 110 mg/dL proposed in the study by Van den Berghe and colleagues and subsequently rapidly generalized to each perioperative patient may be too stringent. Even those who endorse intensive glycemic control disagree regarding the appropriate target glucose level. The discord seems natural because increasingly tight control results in increased risk of hypoglycemia.[61] Although the target BG in the Van den Berghe trial was 80 to 110 mg/dL, a post hoc analysis of the study's results showed reduced morbidity and mortality with decreasing BG levels for surgical patients in ICUs.[37] A study by Golden and colleagues[14] examined several different categories of glucose target (121–26 mg/dL, 207–229 mg/dL, 230–252 mg/dL, and 253–352 mg/dL) and they associated progressively increased infection risk with the 2 highest groups. In addition, a retrospective analysis showed increased hospital mortality with hyperglycemia.[39]

Although the ideal BG target is uncertain, this does not imply that glycemic control should be abandoned. Some investigators have been able to show significant benefit with a target of less than 140 mg/dL[40] and others have shown improved mortality with decreased BG variability.[78,79] Acute fluctuations in BG level have been shown to have detrimental physiologic effects in addition to those of chronic hyperglycemia.[80]

However, these studies are retrospective and lack sufficient data to provide an optimal variability in BG.

There is growing concern over the weight of risk versus benefit with intensive glycemic control. When examining patients from a prospective database and matching them with the control patients from the Van den Berghe study, Egi and colleagues[81] found that the number needed to treat (NNT) was between 38 and 125, whereas the number needed to harm ranged between 7 and 13 depending on the institution. The discrepancy between frequency of benefit as well as frequency of harm is significant even though the potential benefit and harm may not be equivalent, which suggests that the benefit may not be ubiquitous and is not free from complications.

BG MEASUREMENT AND IMPLEMENTATION OF GLYCEMIC CONTROL

In addition to conflicting results over potential outcome benefit and possible harm, disagreement exists over how to measure BG. There are a variety of modalities available for use. The Van den Berghe trial used whole undiluted blood with a blood gas analyzer.[33,44] Many ICUs use point-of-care glucometers that test capillary blood.

The accuracy of these different modalities may vary significantly. Desachy and colleagues[82] compared the accuracy of point-of-care (POC) samples of capillary and whole blood with laboratory values. Their results showed that POC values varied by greater than 20% from laboratory measurements 15% of the time for capillary samples and half that for whole blood samples. In addition, the accuracy of capillary blood values is affected by shock states, low hemoglobin, and hypothermia. Anemia results in a larger plasma volume and hence a greater volume in which glucose is dissolved, falsely increasing POC measurements. In addition, before extraction, arterial BG levels are higher than those in venous or capillary blood.

Another study by Kanji and colleagues[83,84] discovered that consistency between POC values and laboratory measurements was less than 80%, that accuracy dwindled with greater degrees of hypoglycemia, and that false values tended to overestimate the true BG level. This variability makes insulin dosing errors more likely in critically ill individuals, and implies that education regarding glucose measuring devices is essential to safe and effective care, especially in an intensive glycemic control setting.

Device education is just 1 aspect in the complex entity of intensive perioperative glycemic control. By nature, this methodology is resource intensive, requiring significant time, personnel, and quality-controlled equipment. Because of potential variability in skin perfusion owing to shock, hypothermia, and so forth, the subcutaneous route of administration is not preferable in the perioperative and critical care settings. In addition, these formulations tend toward a slower onset than is necessary.[82] According to a recent systematic review, intravenous insulin infusion seems preferable in the setting of a dynamic scale protocol that uses narrow glucose targets, frequent (hourly to every 4 hours) BG checks, as well as the last 2 BG values.[84] This scenario provided the best glycemic control to stated target values with avoidance of hypoglycemia. Protocols would best be designed by those functioning in the perioperative area or critical care unit, those who have nuanced information regarding the intricacies of the patient populations for whom they care; 1 size does not fit all.

SUMMARY AND FUTURE OPTIONS

Early observations of a connection between perioperative hyperglycemia and potential adverse perioperative outcomes evolved into testing the hypothesis that intensive glycemic control may offer an outcome benefit to patients in the perioperative and critical care settings. Significant positive results occurring in this process from such studies as the first Van den Berghe trial[33] resulted in swift acceptance, extrapolation, and application of the potential benefits to heterogeneous patient populations. The Surgical Complications Improvement Project (SCIP) generated by the Joint Commission and Centers for Medicare and Medicaid Services has, possibly prematurely, included perioperative glycemic control in the infection portion of its process and outcome measurements.

Perioperative hyperglycemia may result from a myriad of causes including stress-induced neuroendocrine changes, infection, exogenous glucose administration, and a patient's underlying metabolic state. Moreover, perioperative hyperglycemia is connected to potential adverse outcomes independently of its cause. Because the causes are diverse, so are the patient populations to which intensive glycemic control has been applied. This heterogeneity as well as that of glucose targets and measurement protocols in the several studies has left a variety of questions unanswered (ie, what is most appropriate BG target and to which patient population does this target apply?).

Although the data do not support ubiquitous application of intensive perioperative glycemic control (BG target 80–110 mg/dL), neither should the resultant ambiguity imply that glycemic control be abandoned altogether. It is reasonable to adopt a stance of cautious implementation of an insulin protocol with a BG target such as less than 150 mg/dL importing benefit to some patient populations while avoiding the 3- fold to-6 fold increase in hypoglycemia associated with more intensive strategies. Future technology improving BG measurement and insulin delivery may result in more reliable implementation of intensive glycemic control and thus impart outcome benefit to certain patient populations.

REFERENCES

1. Inzucchi SE. Clinical practice. Management of hyperglycemia in the hospital setting. N Engl J Med 2006;355:1903–11.
2. American Diabetes Association. Standards of medical care in diabetes—2009. Diabetes Care 2009;32(Suppl 1):S13–61.
3. Cowie CC, Rust KF, Ford ES, et al. Full accounting of diabetes and pre-diabetes in the U.S. population in 1988-1994 and 2005-2006. Diabetes Care 2009;32: 287–94.
4. Fahy BG, Sheehy AM, Coursin DB. Glucose control in the intensive care unit. Crit Care Med 2009;37:1769–76.
5. Hertzer NR, Bena JF, Karafa MT. A personal experience with the influence of diabetes and other factors on the outcome of infrainguinal bypass grafts for occlusive disease. J Vasc Surg 2007;46:271–9.
6. Bagry HS, Raghavendran S, Carli F. Metabolic syndrome and insulin resistance: perioperative considerations. Anesthesiology 2008;108:506–23.
7. Puskas F, Grocott HP, White WD, et al. Intraoperative hyperglycemia and cognitive decline after CABG. Ann Thorac Surg 2007;84:1467–73.
8. Bochicchio GV, Sung J, Joshi M, et al. Persistent hyperglycemia is predictive of outcome in critically ill trauma patients. J Trauma 2005;58:921–4.
9. Bochicchio GV, Salzano L, Joshi M, et al. Admission preoperative glucose is predictive of morbidity and mortality in trauma patients who require immediate operative intervention. Am Surg 2005;71:171–4.
10. The UK Prospective Diabetes Study (UKPDS) Group. Intensive blood-glucose control with sulfonylureas or insulin compared with conventional treatment and risk of complications in patients with type 2 diabetes (UKPDS 33). Lancet 1998;352:837–53.

11. Fietsam R, Bassett J, Glover JL. Complications of coronary artery surgery in diabetic patients. Am Surg 1991;57:551–7.
12. Zerr KJ, Fumary AP, Grunkemeier GL, et al. Glucose control lowers the risk of wound infection in diabetics after open-heart operations. Ann Thorac Surg 1997;63(2):356–61.
13. Pomposelli JJ, Baxter JK, Babineau TJ, et al. Early postoperative glucose control predicts nosocomial infection rate in diabetic patients. JPEN J Parenter Enteral Nutr 1998;22:77–81.
14. Golden SH, Peart-Vigilance C, Kao WH, et al. Perioperative glycemic control and the risk of infectious complications in a cohort of adults with diabetes. Diabetes Care 1999;22:1408–14.
15. Furnary AP, Zerr KJ, Grunkemeier GL, et al. Continuous intravenous insulin infusion reduces the incidence of deep sternal wound infection in diabetic patients after cardiac surgical procedures. Ann Thorac Surg 1999;67:352–62.
16. Trick WE, Scheckler WE, Tokars JE, et al. Modifiable risk factors associated with deep sternal site infection after coronary artery bypass grafting. J Thorac Cardiovasc Surg 2000;119:108–14.
17. Trick WE, Scheckler WE, Tokars JE, et al. Risk factors for radial artery harvest site infection following coronary artery bypass graft surgery. Clin Infect Dis 2000;30:270–5.
18. Latham R, Lancaster AD, Covington JF, et al. The association of diabetes and glucose control with surgical- site infections among cardiothoracic surgery patients. Infect Control Hosp Epidemiol 2001;22:607–12.
19. Estrada CA, Young JA, Nifong LW, et al. Outcomes and perioperative hyperglycemia in patients with or without diabetes mellitus undergoing coronary artery bypass grafting. Ann Thorac Surg 2003;75:1932–9.
20. Wheat LJ. Infection and diabetes mellitus. Diabetes Care 1980;3:187–97.
21. Khaodhiar L, McCowen K, Bistrian B. Perioperative hyperglycemia, infection or risk? Curr Opin Clin Nutr Metab Care 1999;2:79–82.
22. Rayfield EJ, Ault MJ, Keusch GT, et al. Infection and diabetes: the case for glucose control. Am J Med 1982;72:439–50.
23. Alexiewicz JM, Kumar D, Smogorzewski M, et al. Polymorphonuclear leukocytes in non-insulin-dependent diabetes mellitus: abnormalities in metabolism and function. Ann Intern Med 1995;123:919–24.
24. Bagdade JD, Root RK, Bulger RJ. Impaired leukocyte function in patients with poorly controlled diabetes. Diabetes 1974;23:9–15.
25. Wilson RM. Neutrophil function in diabetes. Diabet Med 1986;3:509–12.
26. Browne JA, Cook C, Pietrobon R, et al. Diabetes and early postoperative outcomes following lumbar fusion. Spine 2007;32:2214–9.
27. Perner A, Nielsen SE, Rask-Madsen J. High glucose impairs superoxide production from isolated blood neutrophils. Intensive Care Med 2003;29:642–5.
28. Noordzij PG, Boersma E, Schreiner F, et al. Increased preoperative glucose levels are associated with perioperative mortality in patients undergoing noncardiac, nonvascular surgery. Eur J Endocrinol 2007;156:137–42.
29. Yendamuri S, Fulda GJ, Tinkoff GH. Admission hyperglycemia as a prognostic indicator in trauma. J Trauma 2003;55:33–8.
30. Umpierrez GE, Isaacs SD, Bazargan N, et al. Hyperglycemia: an independent marker of in-hospital mortality in patients with undiagnosed diabetes. J Clin Endocrinol Metab 2002;87:978–82.
31. McGirt MJ, Woodworm GF, Brooke BS, et al. Hyperglycemia independently increases the risk of perioperative stroke, myocardial infarction, and death after carotid endarterectomy. Neurosurgery 2006;58:1066–73.

32. Van den Berghe G, Wouters P, Weekers F, et al. Intensive insulin therapy in the critically ill patients. N Engl J Med 2001;345:1359–67.

33. Ouattara A, Lecomte P, Le Manach Y, et al. Poor intraoperative blood glucose control is associated with a worsened hospital outcome after cardiac surgery in diabetic patients. Anesthesiology 2005;103:687–94.

34. Gandhi GY, Nuttall GA, Abel MD, et al. Intraoperative hyperglycemia and perioperative outcomes in cardiac surgery patients. Mayo Clin Proc 2005;80:862–6.

35. Doenst T, Wijcysundera D, Karkouti K, et al. Hyperglycemia during cardiopulmonary bypass is an independent risk factor for mortality in patients undergoing cardiac surgery. J Thorac Cardiovasc Surg 2005;130. 1144.el–1144.e8.

36. Van den Berghe G, Wouters PJ, Bouillon R, et al. Outcome benefit of intensive insulin therapy in critically ill patients: insulin dose versus glycemic control. Crit Care Med 2003;31(3):59–66.

37. Finney SJ, Zekveld C, Elia A, et al. Glucose control and mortality in critically ill patients. JAMA 2003;290:2041–7.

38. Krinsley JS. Association between hyperglycemia and increased hospital mortality in a heterogeneous population of critically ill patients. Mayo Clin Proc 2003;78:1471–8.

39. Krinsley JS. Effect of an intensive glucose management protocol on the mortality of critically ill adult patients. Mayo Clin Proc 2004;79:992–1000.

40. Hansen TK, Thiel S, Wouters PJ, et al. Intensive insulin therapy exerts anti-inflammatory effects in critically ill patients and counteracts the adverse effect of low mannose-binding lectin levels. J Clin Endocrinol Metab 2003;88:1082–8.

41. Weekers F, Giulietti A, Michalaki M, et al. Metabolic, endocrine, and immune effects of stress hyperglycemia in a rabbit model of prolonged critical illness. Endocrinology 2003;144:5329–38.

42. Groeneveld AB, Beinshuizen A, Visser FC. Insulin: a wonder drug in the critically ill? Crit Care 2002;6:102–5.

43. Van den Berghe G, Wilmer A, Hermans G, et al. Intensive insulin therapy in the medical ICU. N Engl J Med 2006;354:449–61.

44. Brunkhorst FM, Engel C, Bloos F, et al, German Competence Network Sepsis (Sep- Net). Intensive insulin therapy and pentastarch resuscitation in severe sepsis. N Engl J Med 2008;358:125–39.

45. Preiser JC. Restoring normoglycaemia: not so harmless. Crit Care 2008;12:116.

46. Gandhi GY, Nuttall GA, Abel MD, et al. Intensive intraoperative insulin therapy versus conventional glucose management during cardiac surgery: a randomized trial. Ann Intern Med 2007;146:233–43.

47. Knapke CM, Owens JP, Mirtallo JM. Management of glucose abnormalities in patients receiving total parenteral nutrition. Clin Pharm 1989;8:136–44.

48. Mizock BA. Alterations in fuel metabolism in critical illness: hyperglycemia. Best Pract Res Clin Endocrinol Metab 2001;15:533–51.

49. Wolfe RR. Carbohydrate metabolism in critically ill patients: implications for nutritional support. Crit Care Clin 1987;3:ll–24.

50. The ESICM Working Group. Metabolic basis of nutrition in intensive care unit patients: ten critical questions. Intensive Care Med 2002;28:1512–20.

51. Schricker T, Lattermann R, Fiset P, et al. Integrated analysis of protein and glucose metabolism during surgery: effects of anesthesia. J Appl Physiol 2001; 91:2523–30.

52. Thorell A, Efendic S, Gutniak M, et al. Insulin resistance after abdominal surgery. Br J Surg 1994;81:59–63.

53. Clarke RS. The hyperglycaemic response to different types of surgery and anaesthesia. Br J Anaesth 1970;42:45–53.

54. Thorell A, Efendic S, Gutniak M, et al. Development of postoperative insulin resistance is associated with the magnitude of operation. Eur J Surg 1993;159:593–9.
55. Thorell A, Nygren J, Essen P, et al. The metabolic response to cholecystectomy: insulin resistance after open compared with laparoscopic operation. Eur J Surg 1996;162:187–91.
56. Schricker T, Berroth A, Pfeiffer U, et al. Influence of vaginal versus abdominal hysterectomy on perioperative glucose metabolism. Anesth Analg 1996;83:991–5.
57. Rassias AJ. Intraoperative management of hyperglycemia in the cardiac surgical patient. Semin Thorac Cardiovasc Surg 2006;18:330–8.
58. Lipshultz AK, Gropper MA. Perioperative glycemic control: an evidence-based review. Anesthesiology 2009;110:408–21.
59. Vriesendorp TM, van Santen S, DeVries JH, et al. Predisposing factors for hypoglycemia in the intensive care unit. Crit Care Med 2006;34:96–101.
60. Krinsley JS, Grover A. Severe hypoglycemia in critically ill patients: risk factors and outcomes. Crit Care Med 2007;35:2262–7.
61. Preiser JC. Intensive glycemic control in Med-Surg patients (European Glucontrol Trial) [abstract]. In Program and abstracts of the Society of Critical Care Medicine 36th Critical Care Congress. Orlando, February 17–21, 2007.
62. Malmberg K, Ryden L, Hamsten A, et al. Effects of insulin treatment on cause-specific one-year mortality and morbidity in diabetic patients with acute myocardial infarction. DIGAMI study group, diabetes insulin-glucose in acute myocardial infarction. Eur Heart J 1996;17:1337–44.
63. Scott JF, Robinson GM, French JM, et al. Glucose potassium insulin infusions in the treatment of acute stroke patients with mild to moderate hyperglycemia: the glucose insulin in stroke trial (GIST). Stroke 1999;30:793–9.
64. Lazar HL, Philippides G, Fitzgerald C, et al. Glucose-insulin-potassium solutions enhance recovery after urgent coronary artery bypass grafting. J Thorac Cardiovasc Surg 1997;113:354–60 [discussion: 360–2].
65. Rao V, Christakis GT, Weisel RD, et al. The Insulin Cardioplegia Trial: myocardial protection for urgent coronary artery bypass grafting. J Thorac Cardiovasc Surg 2002;123:928–35.
66. Lazar HL, Chipkin S, Philippides G, et al. Glucose-insulin- potassium solutions improve outcomes in diabetics who have coronary artery operations. Ann Thorac Surg 2000;70:145–50.
67. Furnary AP, Wu Y, Bookin SO. Effect of hyperglycemia and continuous intravenous insulin infusions on outcomes of cardiac surgical procedures: the Portland Diabetic Project. Endocr Pract 2004;10(Suppl 2):21–33.
68. Furnary AP, Gao G, Grunkemeier GL, et al. Continuous insulin infusion reduces mortality in patients with diabetes undergoing coronary artery bypass grafting. J Thorac Cardiovasc Surg 2003;125:1007–21.
69. D'Alessandro C, Leprince P, Golmard JL, et al. Strict glycemic control reduces EuroSCORE expected mortality in diabetic patients undergoing myocardial revascularization. J Thorac Cardiovasc Surg 2007;134:29–37.
70. Lazar HL, Chipkin SR, Fitzgerald CA, et al. Tight glycemic control in diabetic coronary artery bypass graft patients improves perioperative outcomes and decreases recurrent ischemic events. Circulation 2004;109:1497–502.
71. Bilotta F, Spinelli A, Giovannini F, et al. The effect of intensive insulin therapy on infection rate, vasospasm, neurologic outcome, and mortality in neurointensive care unit after intracranial aneurysm clipping in patients with acute subarachnoid hemorrhage: a randomized prospective pilot trial. J Neurosurg Anesthesiol 2007; 19:156–60.

72. Bellomo R, Egi M. What is a NICE-SUGAR for patients in the intensive care unit? Mayo Clin Proc 2009;84:400–2.

73. Finfer S, Chittock DR, Su SY, et al. Intensive versus conventional glucose control in critically ill patients. N Engl J Med 2009;360:1283–97.

74. Wiener RS, Wiener DC, Larson RJ. Benefits and risks of tight glucose control in critically ill adults: a meta-analysis. JAMA 2008;300:933–44.

75. Lacherade JC, Jabre P, Bastuji-Garin S, et al. Failure to achieve glycemic control despite intensive insulin therapy in a medical ICU: incidence and influence on ICU mortality. Intensive Care Med 2007;33:814–21.

76. Nasraway SA Jr. Sitting on the horns of a dilemma: avoiding severe hypoglycemia while practicing tight glycemic control. Crit Care Med 2007;35:2435–7.

77. Egi M, Bellomo R, Stachowski E, et al. Variability of blood glucose concentration and short-term mortality in critically ill patients. Anesthesiology 2006;105: 244–52.

78. Ali N, O'Brien J, Dungan K, et al. Glucose variability is independently associated with mortality in patients with sepsis. Crit Care Med 2007;36:A257.

79. Monnier L, Mas E, Ginet C, et al. Activation of oxidative stress by acute glucose fluctuations compared with sustained chronic hyperglycemia in patients with type 2 diabetes. JAMA 2006;295:1681–7.

80. Egi M, Bellomo R, Stachowski E, et al. Intensive insulin therapy in postoperative intensive care unit patients: a decision analysis. Am J Respir Crit Care Med 2006; 173:407–13.

81. Desachy A, Vuagnat AC, Ghazali AD, et al. Accuracy of bedside glucometry in critically ill patients: influence of clinical characteristics and perfusion index. Mayo Clin Proc 2008;83:400–5.

82. Kanji S, Buffie J, Hutton B, et al. Reliability of point-of-care testing for glucose measurement in critically ill adults. Crit Care Med 2005;33:2778–85.

83. Chaney MA, Nikolov MP, Blakeman BP, et al. Attempting to maintain normoglycemia during cardiopulmonary bypass with insulin may initiate postoperative hypoglycemia. Anesth Analg 1999;89:1091–5.

84. Meijering S, Corstjens AM, Tulleken JE, et al. Towards a feasible algorithm for tight glycaemic control in critically ill patients: a systematic review of the literature. Crit Care 2006;10:R19.

85. Guvener M, Pasaoglu I, Demircin M, et al. Perioperative hyperglycemia is a strong correlate of postoperative infection in type II diabetic patients after coronary artery bypass grafting. Endocr J 2002;49:531–7.

86. Van den Berghe G, Wilmer A, Milants I, et al. Intensive insulin therapy in mixed medical/surgical intensive care units: benefit versus harm. Diabetes 2006;55: 3151–9.

87. Toft P, Jorgensen HS, Toennesen E, et al. Intensive insulin therapy to non-cardiac ICU patients: a prospective study. Eur J Anaethesiol 2006;23:705–9.

88. Ingels C, Debaveye Y, Milants I, et al. Strict blood glucose control with insulin during intensive care after cardiac surgery: impact on 4-years survival, dependency on medical care, and quality-of-life. Eur Heart J 2006;27:2716–24.

89. Preiser JC, Devos P, Ruiz-Santana S, et al. A prospective randomised multi-center controlled trial on tight glucose control by intensive insulin therapy in adult intensive care units: the Glucontrol study. Intensive Care Med 2009;35(10): 1738–48.

Anxiolytic Use in the Postoperative Care Unit

W. Scott Jellish, MD, PhD*, Michael O'Rourke, MD

KEYWORDS

- Anxiolytics • Perioperative anxiety • Postoperative care unit • Benzodiazepine

KEY POINTS

- Anxiety occurs frequently in patients throughout the perioperative period.
- Recent evidence suggests that postoperative anxiety may have adverse effects on postoperative outcomes in patients.
- It is therefore important for the perioperative physician to be able to recognize and characterize perioperative anxiety.
- Traditionally, pharmacologic therapies such as benzodiazepines have been the mainstay of treatment for perioperative anxiety. However, these medications can increase the risk of postoperative delirium in patients emerging from anesthesia.

Anxiety is a state of uneasiness and apprehension. The perioperative period is often a time of increased anxiety for patients. Surgical patients have many reasons for anxiety including uncertainty about surgical outcomes, apprehension regarding an anesthetic, or uneasiness with a diagnosis requiring surgical intervention. Anxiety is an adaptive feeling that can be beneficial. It can motivate compliance with medical treatment and prompt patients to seek assistance in the perioperative period.[1] However, anxiety symptoms can also be maladaptive. Heightened anxiety can detract from medical treatment by compromising the objectivity of patients, decreasing their tolerance for medical procedures, and causing a constant need for reassurance. This need for ongoing reassurance can strain the patient's social support system as well as the patient's care team.[1] Avoiding perioperative anxiety can hence improve the perioperative experience of the patient.

Anxiety can be described in terms of both state anxiety and trait anxiety. Trait anxiety indicates an anxious personality disposition.[2] People with high trait anxiety are likely to respond to new situations or change with anxiety. A high level of trait anxiety can make a patient more susceptible to high levels of state anxiety in the perioperative period. State anxiety is another term for situational anxiety. It is a temporary

Department of Anesthesiology, Loyola University Medical Center, 2160 S. First Avenue, Maywood, IL 60153, USA
* Corresponding author.
E-mail address: wjellis@lumc.edu

Anesthesiology Clin 30 (2012) 467–480
http://dx.doi.org/10.1016/j.anclin.2012.07.006   **anesthesiology.theclinics.com**

condition stemming from a specific situation. Anesthesiologists encounter state anxiety frequently in preoperative and postoperative patients. Nearly all patients will exhibit some degree of state anxiety during the perioperative period. Typically, state anxiety rather than trait anxiety is the focus of studies of perioperative anxiety.

A variety of questionnaires exist to measure anxiety, including the State-Trait Anxiety Inventory (STAI), the Depression Anxiety Stress Scales (DASS), and the Beck Anxiety Inventory (BAI). The STAI is a 40-item questionnaire of which 20 items are dedicated to state anxiety and 20 to trait anxiety. Scores range from 20 to 80 each for state and trait anxiety.[3] The STAI has been administered to patients at various times during the perioperative period including preoperative testing clinics, the preoperative holding area, the post-anesthesia care unit (PACU) area, during postoperative hospital stay, and also at home or in physician clinics days to months postoperatively. The state anxiety measurement is generally used to estimate a patient's anxiety at a particular point in the perioperative period. The ability to differentiate state from trait anxiety is a strongpoint of the STAI. A second widely used measure of anxiety is the Depression Anxiety Stress Scales (DASS). The DASS is a 42-item questionnaire with 3 subscales: depression, anxiety, and stress. The ability to differentiate depression symptoms from anxiety symptoms is a strength of the DASS.[4,5] The BAI is a 21-item questionnaire. Similar to the DASS, it does not differentiate state from trait anxiety but does differentiate depression from anxiety.[5]

Although anxiety can occur at any time in the perioperative period, it is most commonly treated preoperatively. Preoperative anxiety can increase perioperative pain scores, increase patient distress, increase intraoperative anesthetic requirements, and decrease patient satisfaction.[6] Benzodiazepines have been the traditional treatment for preoperative anxiety, although alternative pharmacologic agents and behavioral therapy have been suggested.

Postoperative anxiety historically has received less attention than preoperative anxiety. Recognition that anxiety occurs throughout the perioperative period has led to increased interest in identifying and treating anxiety in the postoperative period. Caumo and colleagues[7] identified risk factors for postoperative anxiety in adults who presented for elective surgery. Postoperative anxiety was associated with American Society of Anesthesiologists (ASA) III status, moderate to intense postoperative pain, minor psychiatric disorders, preoperative state anxiety, and negative future perception. The same study also found that neural-block anesthesia, systemic multimodal analgesia, and neuroaxial opioids were protective factors against postoperative anxiety. A similar study in children identified high levels of preoperative state anxiety, presence of moderate to intense postoperative pain, and doses of midazolam less than 0.056 mg/kg as risk factors for postoperative anxiety in pediatric patients.[8] In children, a history of previous surgery reduced the risk of postoperative anxiety. These studies reveal the relationship between postoperative anxiety and experience of pain. In both adults and children, high preoperative anxiety and poor pain control are associated with elevated postoperative anxiety (**Box 1**).

The interconnectedness of anxiety and pain experience in the perioperative period has been well demonstrated. However, it is not clear whether anxiety causes postoperative pain or vice versa. Treatment with midazolam preoperatively has been shown to lower postoperative pain scores and decrease postoperative anxiety.[8] Anxious patients are known to have increased patient-controlled analgesia (PCA) demands postoperatively and to have lower pain thresholds.[3] It is clear that perioperative anxiety and pain experience are related, although the causality between the two has not been fully established.

Perioperative anxiety may influence patient outcomes. Presence of preoperative depression is often evaluated preoperatively in patients scheduled for coronary artery

---

Box 1
Risk and protective factors for postoperative anxiety

Risk Factors for Postoperative Anxiety in Adults

Moderate to intense postoperative pain

Preoperative state anxiety

Higher ASA status

History of smoking

Negative future perception

Minor psychiatric disorders

Protective Factors for Postoperative Anxiety in Adults

Neural-block anesthetic

Systemic multimodal analgesia

Neuraxial opioid use

Risk Factors for Postoperative Anxiety in Children

High levels of preoperative state anxiety

Moderate to intense postoperative pain

Administration of midazolam doses less than 0.056 mg/kg

---

bypass grafting (CABG) as a risk factor for poor postoperative outcomes. Recently, anxiety has also gained interest as a risk factor in CABG patients. Two studies have demonstrated that symptoms of anxiety are associated with increased mortality risk for CABG patients.[9,10] The mechanism through which anxiety causes the increased mortality risk is not known. Preoperative anxiety has also been shown to predict readmissions to the hospital after cardiac surgery, independent of medical covariates.[11] The association between anxiety and postoperative mortality is concerning, and may warrant preoperative evaluation for both depression and anxiety in the future to allow preoperative and perioperative monitoring and treatment of these symptoms.

In nonsurgical patients, a correlation has been established between anxiety symptoms and episodes of atrial fibrillation in patients with a history of paroxysmal atrial fibrillation.[12] Patients with paroxysmal atrial fibrillation who experience anxiety symptoms report decreased quality of life. It is thought that controlling anxiety symptoms may prevent episodes of paroxysmal atrial fibrillation. There are several theories as to how anxiety may cause episodes of atrial fibrillation, although a precise mechanism is not known. One theory suggests that dysregulation of the autonomic nervous system as a result of anxiety may contribute to atrial fibrillation. Emotional stress is thought to cause atrial fibrillation through dysregulation of the autonomic nervous system.[13] A similar mechanism whereby anxiety causes dysregulation of the autonomic nervous system has been proposed. Specifically, reduced parasympathetic and increased sympathetic nervous system activity caused by anxiety have been suggested.[14]

This relationship between anxiety and the autonomic nervous system could be important in postoperative cardiac patients who are at risk for postoperative atrial fibrillation. Postoperative CABG patients are known to experience postoperative anxiety. A recent study demonstrated that postoperative anxiety was associated with increased risk of postoperative atrial fibrillation in CABG patients.[14] Causality was not established between anxiety and postoperative atrial fibrillation, but the relationship was evident. As postoperative atrial fibrillation can increase mortality, increase the risk of stroke, and increase hospital stay and total costs, intervention to prevent perioperative anxiety in the future may be warranted in CABG patients.

There are numerous factors that could predispose a patient to high levels of postoperative anxiety. Perioperative anxiety is influenced by the patient's concern about one's health, uncertainty regarding the future, type of surgery and anesthesia performed and, most importantly, concerns about postoperative discomfort. Preoperative anxiety has been found to correlate with high postoperative anxiety.[15] The anxiety the patient has may adversely affect anesthetic recovery and analgesia requirements. No associations have been observed between postoperative state anxiety and gender, age, years in school, extent of surgery, anesthesia, dose of diazepam, midazolam, and fentanyl, history of cancer, previous surgery, or history of alcoholism. Moderate or intense pain was noted to be a risk factor for high levels of postoperative anxiety. This relationship has been described in other studies,[2,16] but the cause of this anxiety has not been totally elucidated. The perception of pain is associated with a high level of state anxiety, and high preoperative anxiety is a predictor of postoperative pain.[2] As stated previously, neural block anesthesia reduced postoperative anxiety. This type of anesthesia prevents several factors associated with increased anxiety such as increased pain immediately after surgery, prolonged hospital stay, decreased satisfaction with the perioperative experience, increased sympathetic tone with sympathetic adrenal activity, and impaired immune function. Aggressive treatment of pain using systemic multimodal analgesia and neuroaxial analgesia has reduced the level of postoperative anxiety in most patients.

Patients who were more anxious in the preoperative period showed an estimated 2.6 times higher risk of reporting a high level of anxiety in the postoperative period. Preoperative diazepam did not protect patients from postoperative anxiety. This finding is explained by the observation that the second peak of action of diazepam occurs 5 to 6 hours after admission, which may be outside the window of time during which patients are recovered sufficiently from their anesthetic to develop anxiety.[17]

Patients with a history of minor psychiatric disorders presented a higher risk for postoperative anxiety.[8]

It is essential to establish pharmacologic and behavioral interventions to reduce postoperative anxiety in patients who are identified with these problems, because it is not cost effective to take such preventive measures for all patients undergoing surgery. A negative preoperative perception of the future was an independent risk factor for postoperative anxiety, with negative future perception increasing stress. Individuals with a negative affect are more likely to have a lower pain threshold and hence are more likely to report increased pain levels.[18]

Smokers also present with a higher risk of developing postoperative anxiety, likely owing to nicotine levels that become reduced because patients are not allowed to smoke in the hospital. A correlation between higher levels of anxiety and nicotine withdrawal symptoms has been shown in preclinical and clinical studies.[19]

Patients who were ill and had multiple comorbidities as represented by ASA physical status had higher levels of postoperative anxiety. This finding suggests the possibility that the patient's preoperative clinical condition could increase stress and anxiety. A significant relationship has been noted between ASA physical status and anesthetic complication.[20] A relationship between ASA physical status and postoperative anxiety has not yet been conclusively established.

Type of surgery may also be important in increasing the incidence of postoperative anxiety. This factor is particularly relevant for emergency surgery patients, who by the nature of the urgent situation have little time to adjust to the fact that they have a problem and need to undergo surgery.[21] The potential negative after-effects of the surgery, the hospitalization and being in a strange environment, coupled with an unfamiliar roommate and possible numerous hospital procedures, produce a great deal of anxiety and stress. Research has demonstrated that preoperative anxiety is related to fears concerning surgical failure, anesthesia, fear of loss of control, and fear of death. Postoperative anxiety has been found to be related to fears of pain, loss of physical functioning, potential negative effects of surgery on body image, and career problems.[22] Certain sociodemographic characteristics such as age, gender, marital status, and education have been noted to be related to anxiety experienced by patients. Women, young individuals, people with low education levels, and single individuals are more vulnerable to anxiety in the postoperative period.[23] It is expected that patients with a high amount of social support will experience lesser anxiety in comparison with those with a low perception of social support.

In some instances, investigators have attempted to develop a biomarker that could help predict which patients will develop postoperative anxiety. Chromogranin A (CgA) is a 48-kDa acidic glycoprotein that is stored and secreted along with catecholamine by the adrenal medulla and sympathetic nerves. This glycoprotein is found in the saliva and is considered to be a biomarker of the stress response produced by the sympatho-adreno-medullary system.[24] Many believe that the increase in this biomarker during stress could also be used to monitor anxiety levels. Studies by Seki-Nakamura and colleagues,[25] however, could not find a good correlation between state or trait anxiety scores and salivary CgA concentration in patients with breast cancer undergoing breast surgery.

Certain disease states and types of surgical interventions will also lead to differing levels of postoperative anxiety that must be treated. Patients with head and neck cancer often exhibit varying degrees of anxiety and panic after their surgery.[26] The occurrence of the panic attacks and anxiety were notable, and pain that sometimes occurs after radical neck procedures was a main contributor. Cervical discomfort, similar to tightening, probably increases the patient's apprehension immediately after surgery (**Fig. 1**). Apprehension and anxiety produce physical sensations such as palpitations and shortness of breath with feelings of choking.

Anxiety and depression are also noted in patients with digestive cancers, who have anxiety amplified by surgical stress. After the declaration of cancer, patients feel strong

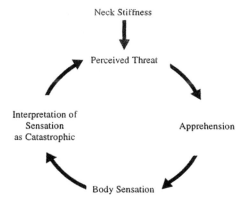

Fig. 1. The panic attack process, as illustrated by a cognitive model of panic. (*Data from* Sist T, Miner M, Lemm AM. Characteristics of post radical neck pain syndrome: a report of 25 cases. J Pain Symptom Manage 1999;18:95–102.)

anxiety for about 2 weeks, but this decreases over time. During treatment the patient feels heightened anxiety that is increased by the surgical procedure. Patients with cancer remain constantly anxious even as the context changes. This anxiety is not ameliorated by changes in the environment. In addition, younger patients are much more anxious than older individuals. Patients with digestive cancer should have effective and well-timed interventions to reduce anxiety immediately after surgery.

Patients with temporal lobe epilepsy undergoing surgery are also known to have high levels of depression with increased state and trait anxiety. The presence of major depression and somatic and psychic anxiety was noted in 15% to 23% of patients after surgery.[27] Anxiety in these patients is high after surgery but gradually decreases over time. Patients experience increased tension and anxiety during the presurgical period because of the anticipation of brain surgery and possible death or neurologic impairment. As time after surgery increases and the patients find they are seizure free without neurologic impairment, their anxiety is significantly reduced.

Patients undergoing cardiopulmonary bypass have also been noted to have more anxiousness than others undergoing different surgical procedures. Many researchers have noted that nocturnal secretion of melatonin from Alzheimer patients, those with coronary artery disease, and stroke patients is decreased.[28] The circadian rhythm of melatonin secretion is disturbed in patients after CABG surgery and cortisol secretion is elevated after these surgeries. The disrupted patterns of melatonin and cortisol secretion in these patients may be correlated directly or indirectly with mood and neuropsychological deficits. Variations in the circadian rhythm of melatonin secretion could result in changes in emotion, perioperative depression, and increased anxiety. Therefore such patients may have an increased predilection for postoperative anxiety because of changes in melatonin and cortisol secretion.

Neurosurgical patients with unruptured intracranial aneurysms have also been noted to have high levels of state anxiety immediately before and after the surgical procedure. State anxiety was reduced later postoperatively, without a change in trait-anxiety scores.[29]

Although certain high-risk patient groups may be more predisposed to postoperative anxiety, almost all postsurgical patients may have some anxiety about the outcome of the surgery or the problems they may have in the immediate postoperative period. Coupled with possible pain, this produces apprehension and anxiety that must be treated to improve patient outcome and recovery. Pharmacologic treatment of postoperative anxiety is by far the major mode of therapy to treat anxiety in the PACU. Traditionally the most widely used anxiolytic-sedative medications are benzodiazepines. With increased dosing, the drugs produce anxiolysis sedation and even unconsciousness. Incremental titration of an intravenous sedative such as diazepam or midazolam can attenuate this psychogenic component. Although diazepam was historically the most commonly used benzodiazepine, midazolam has become the drug of choice because of its short half-life and lack of significant side effects. In fact, several researchers have looked at the use of self-administered midazolam to relieve postoperative anxiety.[16] A PCA pump administering a low dose of midazolam was shown to significantly lower postoperative anxiety in comparison with standard treatments or the use of PCA morphine alone. Lorazepam, because of its long duration of action, is not routinely used for postoperative anxiety. Diazepam may be effective, but again its long half-life and active metabolites may prolong sedation, and prevent patient involvement in postoperative activities such as pulmonary recruitment with deep breathing and early ambulation.

Recovering patients can exhibit inappropriate mental reactions ranging from lethargy and confusion through extreme disorientation and combativeness. Forceful thrashing movements and combative patients can jeopardize suture lines and orthopedic appliances. Agitated, anxious patients manifest high sympathetic tone with tachycardia and hypertension, which can produce medical complications. It is difficult to predict which patients will have emergence reactions. Anxiety in children is undoubtedly heightened by separation from parents. Individuals with mental retardation, clinically evident psychiatric disorders, organic brain dysfunction, or hostile interactions preoperatively have a higher frequency of emergence problems. A language barrier can accentuate emergence reactions and even produce extreme emergence anxiety. Patients premedicated with long-acting sedatives or those taking psychogenic medications can exhibit a clouded sensorium and disorientation. Confusion, delirium, or combativeness after anesthesia can also indicate serious respiratory dysfunction. Moderate hypoxemia often manifests as clouded mentation, disorientation, and agitation, which is difficult to distinguish from pain. Respiratory acidemia caused by airway obstruction or poor ventilation could elicit profound agitation and anxiety. Lactic acidemia from inadequate peripheral perfusion can cause anxiousness and mild disorientation. If cerebral perfusion is not maintained, a patient can exhibit lethargy, disorientation, agitation, and confusion. Metabolic abnormalities interfere with lucidity in the PACU area. Acute hyponatremia or hyperglycemia can cloud consciousness during recovery, with increased anxiety associated with clinical agitation. Once the reversible causes of delirium and anxiety are corrected, the benzodiazepine or other sedative drug can be administered to smooth the emergence. Identifying whether the patient is reacting to pain or anxiety is important when choosing which medication to use. Opioids are relatively poor sedatives, whereas benzodiazepines and barbiturates are poor analgesics. Identifying which to use will help with reducing anxiety by itself or in association with postoperative pain.

Benzodiazepines used for treatment of postoperative anxiety can themselves add to postoperative cognitive dysfunction and delirium, especially in the elderly.[30] Deterioration of memory and concentration has been attributed to benzodiazepines. Hydroxylation of diazepam leads to formation of 3-hydroxydiazepam and demethylation to desmethyldiazepam, which has an elimination half-life of 60 hours. In patients 60 years or older, postoperative cognitive dysfunction was found in 48.6% of patients undergoing abdominal surgery who received diazepam perioperatively. In young patients, a significant correlation was found between plasma concentration of diazepam and slowing of reaction time, but only for a short period (1 hour) after administration. Taken together, postoperative administration of benzodiazepines for possible sedation or anxiolysis could increase the incidence of postoperative cognitive dysfunction for more than a week in elderly patients.

There have been no prospective randomized trials to determine whether certain drugs used in the perioperative period will actually lead to a lowering of postoperative delirium or postoperative cognitive dysfunction. The postoperative use of all benzodiazepines, especially in the elderly, should be avoided if possible, as their use was independently associated with an increased risk of postoperative delirium.[31] The exact mechanism of how benzodiazepines increased delirium is unclear. It is speculated that as these agents have high affinity for the 2-aminobutyric acid receptor in the central nervous system, they may alter levels of neurotransmitters believed to be delirogenic.[32] Benzodiazepines are known to have paradoxic effects such as irritability, aggressiveness, and even confusion. Various reports find more frequent postoperative delirium in the elderly patient on a benzodiazepine. A prospective study by Schor and colleagues,[33] however, found that benzodiazepines were protective for delirium in elderly hospitalized patients, whether for surgery or other reasons. Some other risk factors for postoperative delirium include having breast or abdominal surgery and preoperative use of benzodiazepines. Length of surgery, while possibly additive, had no clinical impact except if exceedingly long. On the other hand, a known history of illness and long-term treatment by antidepressants were found to protect against postoperative delirium, probably because they are themselves anxiolytic and have a long half-life covering the entire length of surgery.

Benzodiazepines in controlled concentrations can also be used to reduce postoperative delirium in elderly patients. Although almost all patients who suffer from postoperative delirium recover in a few days, critical incidents could occur during this delirious state that could lead to severe complications with prolonged hospital time.[31] Many investigators believe that postoperative delirium is related to disorders of the sleep-wake cycle, and attempts have been made to develop a delirium-free protocol. Physicians have used combinations of diazepam, flunitrazepam, and pethidine to maintain a sleep rhythm at night.[34] This approach has been effective for controlling postoperative cognitive dysfunction in elderly patients, with mild morning lethargy as a disadvantage. This artificial control of sleep also has been used to reduce anxiety related to surgery.

Other agents have been noted to reduce postoperative anxiety without the noted side effects of delirium or cognitive dysfunction. Oral gabapentin administered for premedication has been found to improve the quality of and satisfaction with postoperative recovery. Pregabalin, an analogue of gabapentin that possesses anxiolytic, analgesic, and antiepileptic activity, has been shown to be effective in reducing pain and anxiety postoperatively.[35] Pregabalin is alleged to modulate the release of excitatory neurotransmitters, leading to a reduction in levels of anxiety and pain. A study in patients with generalized anxiety disorders found that chronic use of pregabalin was significantly more effective than the benzodiazepine alprazolam in improving anxiety symptoms.[36] However, other studies have found a single dose of preoperative pregabalin to be ineffective in reducing anxiety related to surgery.[37]

Dexmeditomidine has also been shown to be beneficial in reducing anxiety and emergence delirium in the pediatric population. Children with preoperative anxiety have higher excitement scores in the PACU and negative behaviors at home. Furthermore, preoperative anxiety may be linked to emergence delirium.[38] Dexmeditomidine decreased emergence delirium after sevoflurane anesthesia. In addition, subjects receiving dexmeditomidine had less postoperative pain than those receiving midazolam.

Combinations of medications have also been used to reduce postoperative anxiety, especially in children. Midazolam, clonidine, or dexmeditomidine has been administered preoperatively to reduce postoperative pain and anxiety. Premedication with oral midazolam, 0.5 mg/kg, oral clonidine, 4 μg/kg, or transmucosal dexmeditomidine, 1 μg/kg was used to produce postoperative analgesia and reduce anxiety in children. When patients were given α2-agonists before surgery, they had less pain and a tendency toward less sedation after surgery. However, no differences were found in their anxiety scores compared with patients receiving midazolam alone.[39]

Mirtazapine, a nonadrenergic and specific serotonergic antidepressant, is a potent antagonist of central α2 autoreceptors and α2 heteroreceptors, as well as an antagonist of 5-HT$_2$ and 5-HT$_3$ receptors. The 5-HT$_2$ blocking effects contribute to its anxiolytic effects and enhance sleep. Patients given oral disintegrating tablets of mirtazapine 1 hour before surgery had less preoperative anxiety as well as reduced postoperative nausea and anxiety.[40]

Alternative therapies to pharmaceutical treatment of postoperative anxiety have also gained popularity. Acupressure has been shown to be a useful technique for the treatment of pain and anxiety. Kotani and colleagues[41] studied patients scheduled for upper and lower abdominal surgery and reported that intradermal acupuncture increased the proportion of patients experiencing good pain relief with diminished anxiety. Acupressure has also been noted to reduce postoperative anxiety and pain. When individuals are under stress endorphin is released, which elicits interferential obstruction of the pain nerve fiber. When an individual's skin is stimulated by massage or acupressure endorphin levels are increased, which alleviates pain and diminishes anxiety. Ip[42] noted acupressure to have a mean effectiveness rating of 74.4% in alleviating anxiety.

Relaxation techniques have also been used to relieve postoperative pain and anxiety. The therapeutic effects of relaxation can be explained by the theory that anxiety increases muscle tension and then pain. Reducing anxiety and muscle tension by relaxation should also reduce pain. In addition, relaxation is a coping strategy and can help patients feel they have some control over their pain.[43] In orthopedic patients undergoing jaw-relaxation techniques, the pain relief manifested was minimal with no effective reduction in anxiety. This group of patients had a great deal of preoperative pain, and this may have affected the results observed. In patient populations that have minimal or no preoperative pain, relaxation techniques seem to be beneficial.

Massage therapy has also been noted to be beneficial in reducing postoperative pain and anxiety.[44] A pilot study showed that massage therapy can be safely and effectively incorporated into the postoperative care of cardiovascular surgical patients.[45] Pain, anxiety, and tension were decreased in patients who received massage therapy (**Fig. 2**). The decrease in tension and anxiety may be particularly important, given the growing body of evidence showing the worrisome effects of stress on wound healing and immune function. Many pharmacologic interventions targeted to treat pain are fraught with adverse effects that substantially limit their usefulness in many postoperative settings. Massage therapy is nontoxic, safe when provided by experienced therapists, and relatively inexpensive.

Reflexotherapy of the foot has also been shown to relieve both postoperative pain and anxiety in patients with digestive cancers.[46] Reflexology is a manual technique based on the zone theory that reflex points on the foot correspond to organs, glands,

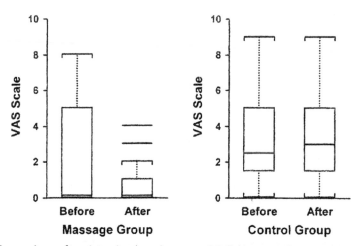

Fig. 2. Comparison of anxiety visual analog score (VAS) between the massage group and the control group before and after intervention. Error bars indicate standard deviation. (*From* Cutshall SM, Wentworth LJ, Engen D, et al. Effect of massage therapy on pain, anxiety, and tension in cardiac surgical patients: a pilot study. Complement Ther Clin Pract 2010;16: 92–5; with permission.)

and parts of the body. When illnesses or imbalances occur in the body, consequent energy channels supposedly become blocked. Reflexology massage is used to open these channels, allowing energy to flow freely. Based on the neuromatrix theory of pain, reflexotherapy is thought to relieve pain by transmitting afferent impulses to close the neural gates in the dorsal horn of the spinal cord.

Reiki is another complementary alternative medicine technique that also has been shown to reduce postoperative pain and anxiety. Reiki is a healing practice that originated thousands of years ago, the term meaning universal life energy. Specific hand positions are learned from Reiki masters to channel life-force energy. These energy-touch therapies all share the subtle effect of moving the human body in the direction of relaxation. In a study using Reiki techniques on women after hysterectomy, the Reiki group demanded much fewer analgesics compared with controls, and state anxiety at discharge was markedly reduced.[47]

Other alternative therapies have also been used to reduce anxiety after surgery. Studies have demonstrated that exposure to calming music can reduce pain and anxiety. There are several positive and negative reports regarding music on perioperative anxiety levels. One study evaluated the use of chair rest with accompanying music and found that patients who listened to music had 72% less anxiety, 57% less pain sensation, and 69% less pain stress than the control group, which experienced chair rest alone.[48] The effects of sedative music may be attributable to having something more pleasant on which to concentrate or something to distract the patient from pain. The use of music for anxiety and pain relief was also attempted with school-age children undergoing same-day surgery.[49] In this patient group, music markedly reduced the need for opiates after surgery and reduced the children's distress scores, but did not seem to reduce anxiety. Children did self report the music as calming and relaxing.

There have been noted benefits of providing information to patients preoperatively concerning their surgery, the procedures they will undergo, and what they must do afterward in reducing postoperative anxiety and stress. Physiotherapy that includes patient assessment, education in procedures to be performed, the relationship such procedures have with breathing capacity, and helping to establish main behaviors postoperatively has been used in cardiac surgery patients, with good results.[50] Using physiotherapy preoperatively reduced anxiety levels in the postoperative period. When patients were educated on ventilatory exercises and hospital routine, anxiety levels decreased when compared with patients without this instruction.

Preoperative instruction has also been successfully used to reduce pain and anxiety after gynecologic surgery.[51] Several studies have noted that anxiety was experienced at a rate of 80% with the fear of not being able to get rid of the cancer and fear of impairment in quality of life producing high levels of anxiety. Also, others have noted that anxiety is increased postoperatively in women who had inaccurate knowledge concerning hysterectomy.[52] By providing an instructional tool about gynecologic surgery and giving patients preoperative preparation, relaxation practice skills, and postoperative self practice for home and clinic, the anxiety felt after surgery was considerably reduced in comparison with those without any preoperative instructions. In addition, for the instructions to be effective in reducing anxiety there was an inverse relation with the patient's education. Patients with higher educational levels had less stress after instruction.

Perioperative dialogue has also been used to reduce stress and anxiety in children.[53] Children who received this dialogue before and after same-day surgery needed significantly less morphine after surgery compared with their counterparts. In one particular study, perioperative dialogue was noted to lower salivary cortisol concentration, which was used as a marker for stress. Salivary cortisol can also be used as a screening tool to find patients who may need better anxiolysis because elevated levels initially could be predictive of higher levels of stress and anxiety. In adolescent children, perioperative dialogue exhibited significantly lower levels of salivary cortisol and lower stress response. To reduce perioperative anxiety, perioperative dialogue, and different steps of caring, continuity and ongoing dialogue by the same anesthesia team serve to complement standard perioperative care.

Guided imagery has also been found to be beneficial as a tool to reduce stress and anxiety. This technique focuses and directs the imagination by mentally engaging all the senses via an imaginal process. Patients may be directed to use imagery for a variety of purposes to regulate mood, revise unhealthy attitudes, and produce coping strategies. It has been helpful in reducing postoperative pain, depression, fatigue, and blood cortisol levels.[54]

This article has outlined the causes of postoperative anxiety, how it is classified, the effects of anxiety on outcomes after surgery, and some of the clinical procedures that produce the highest levels of anxiety for patients. In addition, the authors have attempted to delineate the major risk factors for developing postoperative anxiety as well as classic therapeutic modalities to reduce symptoms and treat the psychological manifestations. Many of the pharmacologic therapies can also increase the risk of postoperative delirium in certain patients emerging from anesthesia, and it is of benefit to know which patients may be at risk for this problem. In addition, new and novel nonpharmacologic therapies promise to provide the broadest therapeutic resource possible for the identification and treatment of postoperative anxiety in patients recovering from major surgical procedures.

REFERENCES

1. Stoudemire A. Human behavior: an introduction for medical students. In: Brown PJ, editor. Human behavior: an introduction for medical students. Philadelphia: Lippincott; 1994. p. 504–5.
2. Thomas V, Heath M, Rose D, et al. Psychological characteristics and the effectiveness of patient-controlled analgesia. Arch Otolaryngol 1995;74:271–6.
3. Julian L. Measures of anxiety. Arthritis Care Res (Hoboken) 2011;63(S11): S467–72.
4. Crawford JR, Henry JD. The depression anxiety stress scales (DASS): normative data and latent structure in a large non-clinical sample. Br J Clin Psychol 2003; 42:111–31.
5. Lovibond PF, Lovibond SH. The structure of negative emotional states: comparison of the depression anxiety stress scales (DASS) with the Beck Depression and Anxiety Inventories. Behav Res Ther 1995;33(3):335–43.
6. Caumo W, Schmidt AP, Schneider CN, et al. Risk factors for preoperative anxiety in adults. Acta Anaesthesiol Scand 2001;45:298–307.
7. Caumo W, Schmidt AP, Schneider CN, et al. Risk factors for postoperative anxiety in adults. Anaesthesia 2001;56:720–8.
8. Kain ZN, Hofstadter MB, Mayes LC, et al. Midazolam effects on amnesia and anxiety in children. Anesthesiology 2000;93:676–84.
9. Rosenbloom JI, Wellenius GA, Mukamal K, et al. Self-reported anxiety and the risk of clinical events and atherosclerotic progression among patients with coronary artery bypass grafts (CABG). Am Heart J 2009;158(5):867–73.
10. Szekely A, Balog P, Benko E, et al. Anxiety predicts mortality and morbidity after coronary artery and valve surgery-A 4-year follow-up study. Psychosom Med 2007;69:625–31.

11. Tully PJ, Baker RA, Turnbull D, et al. The role of depression and anxiety symptoms in hospital readmissions after cardiac surgery. J Behav Med 2008;31:281–90.

12. Suzuki S, Kasanuki H. The influences of psychosocial aspects and anxiety symptoms on quality of life of patients with arrhythmia: investigation on paroxysmal atrial fibrillation. Int J Behav Med 2004;11(2):104–9.

13. Ziegelstein RC. Acute emotional stress and cardiac arrhythmias. JAMA 2007; 298(3):324–9.

14. Tully PJ, Bennetts JS, Baker RA, et al. Anxiety, depression and stress as risk factors for atrial fibrillation after cardiac surgery. Heart Lung 2011;40:4–11.

15. Caumo W, Broenstrub JC, Fialho L, et al. Risk factors for postoperative anxiety in children. Acta Anaesthesiol Scand 2000;44:782–9.

16. Egan KJ, Ready LB, Welssy M, et al. Self administration of midazolam for postoperative anxiety: a double blind study. Pain 1992;49:3–8.

17. Alport CC, Baker JD, Cooke JF. A rational approach to anaesthetic premedication. Drugs 1989;37:219–28.

18. Watson D, Pennebaker JW. Statistical disposition and genetic base of symptom reporting. In: Skelton JA, Croyle RT, editors. Mental representation in health and illness. New York: Springer-Verlag; 1991. p. 60–84.

19. Moadel AB, Laderberg MS, Ostroff JS. Nicotine dependence and withdrawal in the oncology setting: risk factors for psychiatric comorbidity and treatment non-adherence. Psychooncology 1999;8:264–7.

20. Wolters U, Wolf T, Stutzer H, et al. ASA classification and perioperative variables as predictors of postoperative outcome. Br J Anaesth 1996;77:217–22.

21. Karanci AN, Dirik G. Predictors of pre- and postoperative anxiety in emergency surgery patients. J Psychosom Res 2003;55:363–9.

22. Brown S. Quantitative measurement of anxiety in patients undergoing surgery for renal calculus disease. J Adv Nurs 1990;15:962–70.

23. Well JK, Houma GS, Nowlin WF, et al. Presurgical anxiety and post surgical pain adjustment: effect of a stress inoculation procedure. J Consult Clin Psychol 1986; 54:831–5.

24. Noto Y. The relationship between salivary biomarkers and state trait anxiety inventory score under mental arithmetic stress: a pilot study. Anesth Analg 2005;101:1873–6.

25. Seki-Nakamura K, Maebayashi K, Nasu-Izumi S, et al. Evaluation of anxiety and salivary chromogranin A secretion in women receiving breast conserving surgery followed by radiation therapy. J Radiat Res 2011;52:351–9.

26. Sist T, Miner M, Lemm AM. Characteristics of post radical neck pain syndrome: a report of 25 cases. J Pain Symptom Manage 1999;18:95–102.

27. Meldolesi GN, DiGennaro G, Quarato PP, et al. Changes in depression, anxiety, anger, and personality after resective surgery for drug resistant temporal lobe epilepsy: a 2 year follow-up study. Epilepsy Res 2007;77:22–30.

28. Deniz E, Sahara E, Aksula HE. Nitric oxide synthase inhibition in rats: melatonin reduces blood pressure and ischemia reperfusion-induced infarct size. Scand Cardiovasc J 2006;40:248–52.

29. Kubo Y, Ogasawara K, Kashimora H, et al. Cognitive function and anxiety before and after surgery for asymptomatic unruptured intracranial aneurysms in elderly patients. World Neurosurg 2010;73:350–3.

30. Rasmussen LS, Steentoft A, Rasmussen H, et al. Benzodiazepines and postoperative cognition dysfunction in the elderly. Br J Anaesth 1999;83:585–9.

31. Lipowski ZJ. Delirium in the elderly patient. N Engl J Med 1989;320:578–82.

32. Mihic S, Harris R. Alcohol GABA and the $GABA_A$ receptor. Alcohol Health Res World 1997;21:127–31.

33. Schor JD, Leukoff SE, Lipsitz LA, et al. Risk factors for delirium in hospitalized elderly. JAMA 1992;267:827–31.
34. Aizawa KI, Kanai T, Saikawa Y, et al. A novel approach to the prevention of postoperative delirium in elderly after gastrointestinal surgery. Surg Today 2002;32:310–4.
35. Tiippana EM, Hamunen K, Kontinen VK, et al. Do surgical patients benefit from perioperative gabapentin/pragabalin? A systemic review of efficacy and safety. Anesth Analg 2007;104:1545–56.
36. Rickels K, Pollach MH, Feltnor DE, et al. Pregabalin for treatment of generalized anxiety disorder: a 4 week multi-center double blind placebo controlled trial of pregabalin and alprazolam. Arch Gen Psychiatry 2005;623:1022–30.
37. White PF, Tufanogullani B, Taylor J, et al. The effect of pregabalin on preoperative anxiety and sedation levels: a dose ranging study. Anesth Analg 2009;108(4):1140–5.
38. Kain ZN, Caldwell-Andrews AA, Maranets I, et al. Preoperative anxiety and emergency delirium and postoperative maladaptive behavior. Anesth Analg 2004;99:1648–54.
39. Schmidt AP, Valinetti EA, Bandecira D, et al. Effects of pre anesthetic administration of midazolam, clonidine or dexmeditomidine on postoperative pain and anxiety in children. Paediatr Anaesth 2007;17:667–74.
40. Chen CC, Lin CS, Ko YP. Premedication with mirtazapine reduces preoperative anxiety and postoperative nausea and vomiting. Anesth Analg 2008;106:109–13.
41. Kotani N, Hashimoto H, Sato Y, et al. Preoperative intradermal acupuncture reduces postoperative pain, nausea and vomiting, analgesic requirement and sympathoadrenal responses. Anesthesiology 2001;95:349–56.
42. Ip VH. The use of acupuncture for pain relief in a Chinese hospital clinic. Acupunct Med 1999;17:101–9.
43. Roykulcharoen V, Good M. Systemic relaxation to relieve postoperative pain. J Adv Nurs 2004;48(2):140–8.
44. Cutshall SM, Wentworth LJ, Engen D, et al. Effect of massage therapy on pain, anxiety, and tension in cardiac surgical patients: a pilot study. Complement Ther Clin Pract 2010;16:92–5.
45. Mitchinson AR, Kim HM, Rosenberg JM, et al. Acute postoperative pain management using massage as an adjuvant therapy in a randomized trial. Arch Surg 2007;142:1158–67.
46. Tsay SL, Chen HL, Chen SC, et al. Effects of reflexotherapy on acute postoperative pain and anxiety among patients with digestive cancer. Cancer Nurs 2008;31:109–15.
47. Vitale AT, O'Connor PC. The effect of Reiki on pain and anxiety in women after abdominal hysterectomy. Holist Nurs Pract 2006;20(6):263–72.
48. Voss JA, Good M, Yates B, et al. Sedative music reduces anxiety and pain during chair rest after open heart surgery. Pain 2004;112:197–203.
49. Nilsson S, Kokinsky E, Nilsson U, et al. School-aged children's experience of postoperative music medicine on pain, distress and anxiety. Paediatr Anaesth 2009;19:1184–90.
50. Garbossa A, Maldanez E, Mortari DM, et al. Effects of physiotherapeutic instructions on anxiety of CABG patients. Rev Bras Cir Cardiovasc 2009;24(3):359–66.
51. Pinar G, Kurt A, Gingor T. The efficacy of preoperative instruction in reducing anxiety following gynecologic surgery: a case control study. World J Surg Oncol 2011;9:38–42.
52. Farooqi N. Depression and anxiety in patients undergoing hysterectomy. J Pak Psych Soc 2005;2:13–6.

53. Wennstrom B, Tornhage CJ, Nasic S, et al. The perioperative dialogue reduces postoperative stress in children undergoing day surgery as confirmed by salivary cortisol. Paediatr Anaesth 2011;21:1058–65.
54. McKinney CH, Antoni MH, Kumar M, et al. Effects of guided imagery and music (GIM) therapy on mood and cortisol in healthy adults. Health Psychol 1997;16(4): 390–400.

Management of Postoperative Nausea and Vomiting

How to Deal with Refractory PONV

Johanna Jokinen[a], Andrew F. Smith[b], Norbert Roewer, MD, PhD[a],
Leopold H.J. Eberhart, MD, PhD, MA[c], Peter Kranke, MD, PhD, MBA[a],*

KEYWORDS

- Postoperative nausea and vomiting • PONV • Postoperative complications
- Patient satisfaction • Enhanced recovery • Recovery after anesthesia and surgery

KEY POINTS

- Postoperative nausea and vomiting (PONV) constitutes a significant factor in delaying recovery after anesthesia and impairing patient satisfaction.
- There has been extensive research in the management of PONV showing that aggressive prophylaxis measures, combined with changes in anesthetic technique, can significantly reduce the incidence of PONV.
- Implementation and knowledge transfer of the latest accomplishments in the prevention of PONV is only slowly being adopted into clinical practice.
- Multimodal prevention in conjunction with early and aggressive treatment constitute key elements in reducing the incidence of refractory PONV.

INTRODUCTION

Without prophylaxis, about 30% of patients undergoing general anesthesia are likely to experience postoperative nausea and vomiting (PONV).[1–3] In a patient population with multiple risk factors, the incidence is up to 80%.[3] PONV has a significant negative effect on patient satisfaction with anesthesia[4] and is one of the most common causes for unplanned hospital admissions in day-case surgery.[5] Even though rare, there can be severe complications following PONV, such as Boerhaave syndrome, airway compromise, and emphysema.[6–11] Considering these facts, it should be essential for every anesthesiologist to aim for a PONV-free recovery.[12,13]

Disclosure: P.K. and L.H.J.E. have consulted for ProStrakan, Ltd.
[a] Department of Anaesthesia and Critical Care, University Hospitals of Würzburg, Oberdürrbacher Strasse 6, Würzburg 97080, Germany; [b] Lancaster Patient Safety Research Unit, Royal Lancaster Infirmary, Ashton Road, Lancaster, LA1 4RP, UK; [c] Department of Anaesthesiology and Intensive Care, Philipps-University Marburg, Baldingerstrasse, Marburg D-35033, Germany
* Corresponding author.
E-mail address: Kranke_p@klinik.uni-wuerzburg.de

Anesthesiology Clin 30 (2012) 481–493
http://dx.doi.org/10.1016/j.anclin.2012.07.003   **anesthesiology.theclinics.com**

Such is especially true considering that an adequate prophylaxis decreases the incidence of PONV significantly, with a low risk of potential side effects from antiemetics. Scuderi and colleagues[14] even showed a response rate of 98% in a randomized controlled trial using multimodal management to prevent PONV. Irrespective of the preventive strategy and whether a liberal or restrictive use of antiemetics is applied, the treatment of established PONV should be immediate and effective. A systematic review by Eberhart and colleagues[15] revealed a high recurrence rate of PONV of between 65% and 84% in patients treated with placebo after the first episode of PONV. Thus, a "wait-and-see" strategy cannot be recommended. Rather, it should be considered whether treatment with a single agent is sufficient or whether, in view of a better long-term protection against PONV recurrence,[16] a combined or even multimodal treatment should be instituted.[17]

RISK FACTORS

Apfel and colleagues[3] identified several risk factors for PONV and, among other groups, established a useful simplified risk score as an easy way to assess risk. Risk factors include female gender, history of motion sickness or PONV, nonsmoking status, and the use of postoperative opioids. Other studies found additional factors that may increase the incidence of PONV such as young age, the use of volatile anesthetics, longer duration of anesthesia, and the administration of nitrous oxide.[18] Even if this allows preoperative risk identification, the prediction is not highly accurate, achieving a rate of 55% to 80%.[19] Therefore it is recommended that PONV prophylaxis should be given to every patient or at least to every patient with one or more risk factors. Given that the potential to cause adverse effects with antiemetics is low,[20] and considering the additive effect when multimodal PONV prevention is applied,[21] there is considerable room for improvement, which holds especially true when taking into account that risk-adapted approaches rarely yield a compliance rate that could be considered optimal.[22]

PROPHYLAXIS

Current evidence suggests that prophylaxis should involve different antiemetics and, especially in high-risk patients, general anesthesia without volatile anesthetics or nitrous oxide (**Fig. 1**). The use of 2 or more antiemetics of different groups decreases the risk of PONV more effectively than the use of just one type of antiemetic. Complex multimodal strategies as used in the study of Scuderi and colleagues[14] show a good success rate in preventing PONV and suggest that, providing a multimodal management protocol is applied, PONV should no longer constitute a major problem for virtually all patients. Thus, prophylaxis is the first step in avoiding refractory PONV. However, several publications show difficulties with implementation of guidelines for the prevention of PONV.[23,24] To increase compliance with guidelines, the authors recommend keeping guidelines as simple as possible and to encourage a rather liberal use of prophylactic antiemetics. One option is to give prophylaxis to all patients regardless of the individual risk score and extend this prophylaxis scheme if the patient has a high risk of experiencing PONV, as shown in **Fig. 1**. This approach guarantees that every patient at risk receives at least some kind of prophylaxis. Given that antiemetics are generally cheap and have few side effects, it is reasonable to administer them even to patients with a low risk, to achieve coverage of all patients at higher risk with a good prophylaxis. Such an approach is supported by the fact that individual prediction (deciding whether one specific patient will actually vomit) is rather poor and that in many patient populations, the majority of patients have 2 or more risk factors

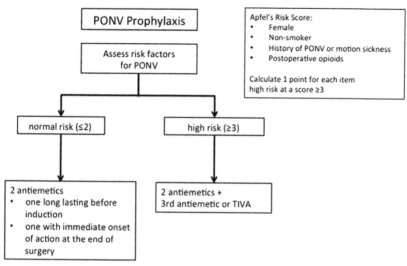

Fig. 1. Algorithm for PONV prophylaxis.

anyway. Another issue remains the ongoing discussion as regards the precise definition of items of risk scores. How should people deal with a patient having suffered from PONV in 1 out of 4 previous anesthetics? Are we dealing with a smoker if a patient admits to smoke once per month? When does motion sickness become motion sickness? And how do we define the dose response of opioids causing PONV when it comes to judging whether this factor (which should be assessed before waking a patient up) is present or not?

TREATMENT OF ESTABLISHED PONV

Established PONV and its treatment have been far less investigated than its prevention.[25] Most trials have analyzed the effect of 5-HT$_3$ receptor antagonists (RAs). There is a lack of evidence for the administration of classic antiemetics in established PONV. Even if widely used in clinical practice, appropriate trials have rarely been conducted. Regarding the pathophysiology of PONV and the use of these antiemetics in situations other than established PONV, it is believed they are efficient in the treatment of PONV as well. Nevertheless, reliable data are lacking.

5-HT$_3$ Receptor Antagonists

The 5-HT$_3$ (serotonin) RAs are the most investigated antiemetics for prophylaxis and treatment of PONV. These agents are highly effective for PONV prevention and treatment. In their systematic review, Kazemi-Kjellberg and colleagues[25] found a number needed to treat (NNT) for 5-HT$_3$ RAs between 2.3 and 4.7 concerning the prevention of further vomiting after established PONV. Between 6 and 24 hours postoperatively, 5-HT$_3$ RAs were less successful in preventing vomiting and the NNT increased to 2.8 to 6.0. Most of the included trials were investigating ondansetron. Other "setrons" may prove as effective as ondansetron. The data obtained with prevention do suggest exactly this. Assumptions that granisetron may be associated with better efficacy[26] should be interpreted with great caution because these results rely on the inclusion of the data compiled by Fujii and colleagues that are currently being investigated and may turn out to be fraudulent.[27–30] No trials were included that investigated the newest 5-HT$_3$ RA, palonosetron. Palonosetron has a longer half-life than ondansetron and other 5-HT$_3$ RAs,[31] and might therefore be more appropriate for the prevention of PONV in the extended postoperative period. It also seems to be more effective for prophylaxis and shows fewer side effects such as headache or QT-interval prolongation.[32–34]

Glucocorticoids

Dexamethasone is an effective drug in preventing PONV. It is a long-lasting agent with delayed onset of action, and should be given before the induction to achieve maximum prophylaxis.[35] However, recent trials also show an effect of dexamethasone in established PONV. Dexamethasone added to other antiemetics with immediate onset of action, such as 5-HT$_3$ antagonists or a dopamine antagonist (haloperidol), significantly decreased the recurrence of PONV.[16,36]

Antihistamines

Antihistamines, such as dimenhydrinate and cyclizine, are commonly used in practice. Nevertheless, the data investigating their effectiveness in established PONV are poor.

There are several studies evaluating their efficiency for prevention, and a meta-analysis showed a risk reduction for PONV.[37] Therefore, they can also be considered for treatment.

Neurokinin-1 Receptor Antagonists

Neurokinin-1 (NK1) RAs are the newest class of antiemetics. Studies focusing on prophylaxis of PONV showed that NK1-RAs are as effective as 5-HT$_3$ antagonists, and more potent in preventing vomiting. Compared with 5-HT$_3$ antagonists, NK1 RAs are not associated with QT prolongation and have a longer half-life (except palonosetron, which has a comparable half-life). Aprepitant is available as an oral formulation and as fosaprepitant, an intravenous prodrug of aprepitant (currently approved by the Food and Drug Administration [FDA] for chemotherapy-induced nausea and vomiting treatment only). The newer NK1 antagonists casopitant and rolapitant have a longer half-life (up to 120 hours) but are not FDA approved. In 2009 the FDA rejected the approval of Casopitant, requesting more data.[38] These agents show encouraging results in the prevention of PONV for the time period up to 120 hours postoperatively.[39–41] As they are the most effective class of antiemetics for the prevention and treatment of vomiting, NK1 RAs should especially be considered for patients with a very high risk for PONV and medical risks associated with vomiting.[42]

Cholinergic Antagonists

An antiemetic with a long-lasting prevention of PONV is transdermal scopolamine. When administered before surgery it prevents PONV significantly for 24 to 48 hours postoperatively. As a cholinergic antagonist, its side effects include dry mouth and visual disturbances.[43] Other possible side effects caused by the inhibition of cholinergic receptors are less likely when used for PONV prophylaxis.[44] Because its onset of action is slow, transdermal scopolamine given for the treatment of PONV should be combined with an antiemetic that acts immediately.

Butyrophenone

Dopamine antagonists such as droperidol reduce PONV, and there have been several trials investigating their effectiveness for treatment.[25] Although they have been found to be effective in treatment and prophylaxis of PONV, there have been reports of cardiac arrhythmias and QT prolongation, which have led to a controversial debate and the issuing of warnings.[45–47] The result is that in the United States patients now require a 12-lead electrocardiogram (ECG) before administration of droperidol and haloperidol, and ECG monitoring for at least 3 hours after their administration,[48] which might limit their use in PONV management on the ward or in postdischarge nausea and vomiting in some countries.[49] Because the availability and experience with these types of drugs on the ward is limited, the investigators suggest the use within licensed indications as preventive measures in the operating room or as treatment in the post-anesthesia care unit (PACU). There is evidence that droperidol at the recommended doses is more potent than the recommended and investigated doses of metoclopramide.[50] Because increasing the dose of these substances leads to more adverse effects,[51] it is reassuring to note that low-dose droperidol is also effective.[52]

Metoclopramide

A meta-analysis in 1999 found no evidence that metoclopramide was effective in preventing nausea, with an NNT of 9.1 for prevention of vomiting.[51] The l'Abbé plot in this important meta-analysis, however, showed that metoclopramide, even at the investigated doses, is better than the placebo with which it was compared, albeit less effective than standard antiemetics, for example, 4 mg ondansetron, 4 mg dexamethasone, or 1 mg droperidol. However, Wallenborn and colleagues[53] found evidence of dose responsiveness; 10 mg, as commonly used in practice and in most trials, did not achieve a significant effect, whereas 25 mg and 50 mg did. Therefore it is recommended to administer 20 to 25 mg metoclopramide, although it slightly increases the risk of side effects such as tachycardia and hypotension. Because a combination of 2 dopamine-2 (D2) antagonists, based on what is known to date, does not make sense, it may be speculated and assumed that it is more reasonable to use droperidol as the D2 antagonist within the anti-PONV armamentarium.

HOW TO USE ANTIEMETICS IN PRACTICE

Basically all antiemetic techniques that are used for preventing PONV can be used for treatment as well, except total intravenous anesthesia (**Table 1, Fig. 2**). Because of their slow onset of action, transdermal scopolamine and dexamethasone should not be considered as first-line treatment of acute nausea and vomiting, but might be indicated as a secondary prevention in the case of PONV.[54] The choice of antiemetics for treatment should depend on local hospital guidelines, patients' medical history (to account for potential contraindications), and agents used in previous prophylaxis. In this context, there is good evidence that repeating the same type of antiemetic in the PACU that has been used for prophylaxis shows no benefit for the patient.[55] Of course, in addition to the choice and administration of antiemetics, possible treatable causes of nausea and vomiting should be considered and excluded. Examples are shown in **Box 1**. However, it should be noted that PONV in most cases is simply PONV, that is, a consequence of triggers that are associated with anesthetic agents, mainly volatile anesthetics and opioids. The exclusion of other factors does play a more important role as the influence of the drugs administered for anesthesia wears off (ie, after 24 hours).

As Franck and colleagues[1] showed, PONV is often undetected by nursing staff in the recovery room or on the ward. Therefore it is important to actively ask the patient at frequent intervals after surgery whether he or she is experiencing PONV. This study also proves that simply relying on treatment and then to aggressively treat PONV

Table 1
Intravenous antiemetic doses for adults and children

Group	Drug	Adult Dose (mg)	Child Dose (mg/kg)	Side Effects
5-HT$_3$ receptor antagonists	Ondansetron	4	0.1	Headache, obstipation, elevated transaminases, QT prolongation
	Dolasetron	12.5	0.35	There are no side effects known yet for Palonosetron
	Tropisetron	2	0.1	
	Granisetron	1	0.02	
	Palonosetron	0.075		
NK1 receptor antagonists	Aprepitant	40 (by mouth)		Headache, obstipation, elevated transaminases, dry mouth, drowsiness
	Fosaprepitant	115		
Glucocorticoids	Dexamethasone	4–8	0.15	Hypotension, reflexive tachycardia, hypertension, increases blood sugar
Antihistamines	Dimenhydrinate	62	0.5	Drowsiness, dry mouth, tachycardia, QT prolongation, visual disturbances, dysuria
	Cyclizine	50		
Cholinergic antagonists	Scopolamine	1 per 24 h (transdermal)		Visual disturbances, dry mouth, confusion, hallucinations
Butyrophenone	Droperidol	0.625–1.25	0.01	QT prolongation, hypotension, reflexive tachycardia, drowsiness, dystonia, anxiety
	Haloperidol	1–2		Agitation, insomnia, akathisia, dyskinesia, headache, hypotension, dry mouth, visual disturbances, QT prolongation
Benzamide	Metoclopramide	25		Hypotension, reflexive tachycardia, dyskinesia

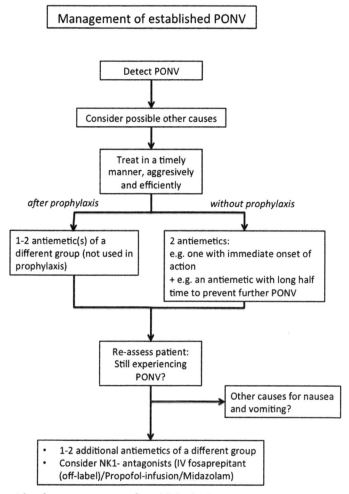

| Management of established PONV |

Detect PONV

↓

Consider possible other causes

↓

Treat in a timely manner, aggresively and efficiently

after prophylaxis   *without prophylaxis*

1-2 antiemetic(s) of a different group (not used in prophylaxis)

2 antiemetics:
e.g. one with immediate onset of action
+ e.g. an antiemetic with long half time to prevent further PONV

↓

Re-assess patient: Still experiencing PONV?

Other causes for nausea and vomiting?

↓

• 1-2 additional antiemetics of a different group
• Consider NK1- antagonists (IV fosaprepitant (off-label)/Propofol-infusion/Midazolam)

Fig. 2. Algorithm for management of established PONV.

should it occur has to be considered suboptimal in most clinical settings. Lack of awareness that PONV constitutes a relevant issue for patients makes it unlikely that PONV is detected early and aggressively treated.

TREATMENT AFTER PROPHYLAXIS

If PONV occurs in a patient despite having received prophylaxis, the antiemetic of choice should belong to a different class of drug to the ones previously given.[56] Because different antiemetic groups act through different mechanisms, the rescue drug should affect another receptor class to achieve additional effects. Moreover, an antiemetic might be ineffective if used as prophylaxis before; for example, ondansetron given as prophylaxis and again for treatment within 2 hours postoperatively had no convincing additive effect.[57] Although there is no good evidence from randomized controlled trials, there is good reason to assume that the same holds true for other antiemetic classes.[55]

Box 1
Possible causes of PONV

- Pain
- Hypotension
- Hypoxia
- Drugs
- Gastrointestinal abnormality (ileus etc)
- Unnecessary nasogastric tube
- Mobilization
- Increased eye pressure (acute glaucoma)

COMBINATIONS OF ANTIEMETICS

The additive effect of antiemetics used in combination for prophylaxis has been well investigated. There is some evidence of additive effects in treatment of established PONV also. Dexamethasone in combination with either dolasetron, haloperidol, ondansetron, or droperidol has been associated with an increase of the antiemetic effect in different trials.[16,36] It might be useful to combine antiemetics that have an immediate onset of action (eg, 5-HT$_3$ RA or low-dose droperidol) with antiemetics that have a long half-life (eg, dexamethasone, scopolamine, NK1 RAs) to obtain immediate successful relief of PONV and prevention of recurrence for as long as possible. Patient care on the ward typically is less intense than in the PACU, and the detection of PONV and timely treatment on the ward may turn out to be more difficult to achieve than in the PACU.[1]

OTHER OPTIONS TO TREAT PONV
Propofol

The findings of the antiemetic effect of propofol are inconsistent and seem to be dose related. There is some evidence that propofol infusion prevents PONV during administration and that it can be helpful in refractory PONV.[58] However, propofol given in an effective dose can cause sedation and is therefore only an option when the patient can be monitored adequately. Propofol has been used with a patient-controlled mode[59] and turned out to be effective in chemotherapy-induced nausea and vomiting.[60] Long-term effects are lacking and if PONV persists, the presumably unspecific sedative effects in the vomiting centers should be substituted with other agents, such as midazolam, given in low doses.

Acupressure

Several trials and reviews have investigated the effect of acupressure at the P6 acupoint for prophylaxis. It is a nondrug option to decrease the incidence of PONV, with minor side effects. The relative risk for PONV in a Cochrane Review with meta-analysis was about 0.7.[61] It therefore may be offered to patients as additional treatment if the placement on the patient's wrist is possible, and may turn out to be a useful intervention if the risk-to-benefit assessment suggests a more cautious use of prophylactic antiemetics, for example, during breastfeeding or pregnancy.

Inhalation of Isopropyl Alcohol

The findings of whether the inhalation of isopropyl alcohol decreases the incidence of PONV are inconsistent. Some studies report it as an effective procedure,[62,63] whereas others found no effect or even an increase of the occurrence of PONV.[64,65] Overall, the methodological quality of the existing studies is not as good as with pharmacologic management, which is especially true for the long-term effects (ie, efficacy over 24 hours), so this option cannot be recommended on the basis of evidence.

SUMMARY

Having a high recurrence rate, established PONV should be treated immediately, aggressively, and effectively using a multimodal approach. Even though all antiemetic classes can be used for the treatment of PONV, 5-HT$_3$ RAs are the best investigated antiemetics to date. With an NNT between 2.3 and 4.7, they can effectively prevent further vomiting. Palonosetron, a new 5-HT$_3$ RA, shows benefits deriving from its longer half-life and fewer side effects. NK1 RAs have also been shown to be very effective, in fact being the most effective currently available class of drugs for vomiting. Thus for patients suffering from refractory vomiting, NK1 RAs might in the future be the key to treatment. However, thus far there are no preparations licensed for intravenous use. Moreover, to date there is no evidence that drugs effective in prevention may not be equally effective in treatment. The challenges with treatment are (1) to ensure that relief is guaranteed quickly, and (2) that nausea is recognized as the most important aspect of PONV. Therefore if patients are not asked about the occurrence of PONV, there is a high chance that it will be missed, both in the PACU and on the ward. If PONV becomes refractory to the drugs already given, a bolus of propofol (10–20 mg, given repeatedly) may turn out to be a useful rescue option. If this works, a continuous infusion of propofol can be tried, even though the supporting data are inconsistent. Repetition of substances given as prevention or treatment may be considered for the short-acting interventions (eg, ondansetron), after 6 hours following the initial dose. However, useful data regarding the latter question are sparse. As for prophylaxis, it is more effective to combine antiemetics of different classes to achieve better treatment of established PONV. The chosen antiemetics should belong to a class other than the ones used for prevention. Nevertheless, the data for treatment of PONV are poor, as most trials have investigated their use in prophylaxis. Although the prevention of PONV is among the most widely investigated clinical problems in conjunction with anesthesia, further studies are needed to define the optimal treatment of established PONV, which is still underrepresented in existing clinical trials.

REFERENCES

1. Franck M, Radtke FM, Apfel CC, et al. Documentation of post-operative nausea and vomiting in routine clinical practice. J Int Med Res 2010;38(3):1034–41.
2. Cohen MM, Duncan PG, DeBoer DP, et al. The postoperative interview: assessing risk factors for nausea and vomiting. Anesth Analg 1994;78(1):7–16.
3. Apfel CC, Laara E, Koivuranta M, et al. A simplified risk score for predicting post-operative nausea and vomiting: conclusions from cross-validations between two centers. Anesthesiology 1999;91(3):693–700.
4. Eberhart LH, Morin AM, Wulf H, et al. Patient preferences for immediate postoperative recovery. Br J Anaesth 2002;89(5):760–1.
5. Blacoe DA, Cunning E, Bell G. Paediatric day-case surgery: an audit of unplanned hospital admission Royal Hospital for Sick Children, Glasgow. Anaesthesia 2008; 63(6):610–5.
6. Schumann R, Polaner DM. Massive subcutaneous emphysema and sudden airway compromise after postoperative vomiting. Anesth Analg 1999;89(3):796–7.

7. Baric A. Oesophageal rupture in a patient with postoperative nausea and vomiting. Anaesth Intensive Care 2000;28(3):325–7.

8. Atallah FN, Riu BM, Nguyen LB, et al. Boerhaave's syndrome after postoperative vomiting. Anesth Analg 2004;98(4):1164–6.

9. Bremner WG, Kumar CM. Delayed surgical emphysema, pneumomediastinum and bilateral pneumothoraces after postoperative vomiting. Br J Anaesth 1993; 71(2):296–7.

10. Reddy S, Butt MW, Samra GS. A potentially fatal complication of postoperative vomiting: Boerhaave's syndrome. Eur J Anaesthesiol 2008;25(3):257–9.

11. Toprak V, Keles GT, Kaygisiz Z, et al. Subcutaneous emphysema following severe vomiting after emerging from general anesthesia. Acta Anaesthesiol Scand 2004; 48(7):917–8.

12. Kranke P, Eberhart LH. Possibilities and limitations in the pharmacological management of postoperative nausea and vomiting. Eur J Anaesthesiol 2011; 28(11):758–65.

13. Kranke P, Schnabel A, Eberhart LH, et al. Providing effective implementation of antiemetic strategies: the postoperative nausea and vomiting-free hospital is a laudable and realistic goal. Eur J Anaesthesiol 2011;28(4):308–9.

14. Scuderi PE, James RL, Harris L, et al. Multimodal antiemetic management prevents early postoperative vomiting after outpatient laparoscopy. Anesth Analg 2000;91(6):1408–14.

15. Eberhart LH, Frank S, Lange H, et al. Systematic review on the recurrence of postoperative nausea and vomiting after a first episode in the recovery room: implications for the treatment of PONV and related clinical trials. BMC Anesthesiol 2006;6:14.

16. Rusch D, Arndt C, Martin H, et al. The addition of dexamethasone to dolasetron or haloperidol for treatment of established postoperative nausea and vomiting. Anaesthesia 2007;62(8):810–7.

17. Tramer MR. Rational control of PONV—the rule of three. Can J Anaesth 2004; 51(4):283–5.

18. Leslie K, Myles PS, Chan MT, et al. Risk factors for severe postoperative nausea and vomiting in a randomized trial of nitrous oxide-based vs nitrous oxide-free anaesthesia. Br J Anaesth 2008;101(4):498–505.

19. Gan TJ. Risk factors for postoperative nausea and vomiting. Anesth Analg 2006; 102(6):1884–98.

20. Carlisle JB, Stevenson CA. Drugs for preventing postoperative nausea and vomiting. Cochrane Database Syst Rev 2006;(3):CD004125.

21. Apfel CC, Korttila K, Abdalla M, et al. A factorial trial of six interventions for the prevention of postoperative nausea and vomiting. N Engl J Med 2004;350(24): 2441–51.

22. Franck M, Radtke FM, Baumeyer A, et al. Adherence to treatment guidelines for postoperative nausea and vomiting. How well does knowledge transfer result in improved clinical care? Anaesthesist 2010;59(6):524–8 [in German].

23. Kooij FO, Klok T, Hollmann MW, et al. Decision support increases guideline adherence for prescribing postoperative nausea and vomiting prophylaxis. Anesth Analg 2008;106(3):893–8.

24. Frenzel JC, Kee SS, Ensor JE, et al. Ongoing provision of individual clinician performance data improves practice behavior. Anesth Analg 2010;111(2):515–9.

25. Kazemi-Kjellberg F, Henzi I, Tramer MR. Treatment of established postoperative nausea and vomiting: a quantitative systematic review. BMC Anesthesiol 2001; 1(1):2.

26. Tang DH, Malone DC. A network meta-analysis on the efficacy of serotonin type 3 receptor antagonists used in adults during the first 24 hours for postoperative nausea and vomiting prophylaxis. Clin Ther 2012;34(2):282–94.

27. Carlisle JB. A meta-analysis of prevention of postoperative nausea and vomiting: randomised controlled trials by Fujii et al. compared with other authors. Anaesthesia 2012, in press.

28. Kranke P, Apfel CC, Eberhart LH, et al. The influence of a dominating centre on a quantitative systematic review of granisetron for preventing postoperative nausea and vomiting. Acta Anaesthesiol Scand 2001;45(6):659–70.

29. Kranke P, Apfel CC, Roewer N, et al. Reported data on granisetron and postoperative nausea and vomiting by Fujii, et al. are incredibly nice! Anesth Analg 2000;90(4):1004–7.

30. Kranke P, Wallenborn J, Roewer N, et al. Fraud or flawed? at the end of the day it may be the patient who pays the bill! Clin Ther 2012;34(5):1204–6 [author reply: 1206–8].

31. Wong EH, Clark R, Leung E, et al. The interaction of RS 25259-197, a potent and selective antagonist, with 5-HT3 receptors, in vitro. Br J Pharmacol 1995;114(4): 851–9.

32. Bajwa SS, Bajwa SK, Kaur J, et al. Palonosetron: a novel approach to control postoperative nausea and vomiting in day care surgery. Saudi J Anaesth 2011; 5(1):19–24.

33. Melton MS, Klein SM, Gan TJ. Management of postdischarge nausea and vomiting after ambulatory surgery. Curr Opin Anaesthesiol 2011;24(6):612–9.

34. Park SK, Cho EJ. A randomized, double-blind trial of palonosetron compared with ondansetron in preventing postoperative nausea and vomiting after gynaecological laparoscopic surgery. J Int Med Res 2011;39(2):399–407.

35. Wang JJ, Ho ST, Tzeng JI, et al. The effect of timing of dexamethasone administration on its efficacy as a prophylactic antiemetic for postoperative nausea and vomiting. Anesth Analg 2000;91(1):136–9.

36. Ormel G, Romundstad L, Lambert-Jensen P, et al. Dexamethasone has additive effect when combined with ondansetron and droperidol for treatment of established PONV. Acta Anaesthesiol Scand 2011;55(10):1196–205.

37. Kranke P, Morin AM, Roewer N, et al. Dimenhydrinate for prophylaxis of postoperative nausea and vomiting: a meta-analysis of randomized controlled trials. Acta Anaesthesiol Scand 2002;46(3):238–44.

38. Available at: http://www.ukmi.nhs.uk/applications/ndo/record_view_open.asp?new DrugID=4373. Accessed September 7, 2012.

39. Singla NK, Singla SK, Chung F, et al. Phase II study to evaluate the safety and efficacy of the oral neurokinin-1 receptor antagonist casopitant (GW679769) administered with ondansetron for the prevention of postoperative and postdischarge nausea and vomiting in high-risk patients. Anesthesiology 2010; 113(1):74–82.

40. Altorjay A, Melson T, Chinachoit T, et al. Casopitant and ondansetron for postoperative nausea and vomiting prevention in women at high risk for emesis: a phase 3 study. Arch Surg 2011;146(2):201–6.

41. Gan TJ, Gu J, Singla N, et al. Rolapitant for the prevention of postoperative nausea and vomiting: a prospective, double-blinded, placebo-controlled randomized trial. Anesth Analg 2011;112(4):804–12.

42. Apfel CC, Malhotra A, Leslie JB. The role of neurokinin-1 receptor antagonists for the management of postoperative nausea and vomiting. Curr Opin Anaesthesiol 2008;21(4):427–32.

43. Kranke P, Morin AM, Roewer N, et al. The efficacy and safety of transdermal scopolamine for the prevention of postoperative nausea and vomiting: a quantitative systematic review. Anesth Analg 2002;95(1):133–43.
44. Apfel CC, Zhang K, George E, et al. Transdermal scopolamine for the prevention of postoperative nausea and vomiting: a systematic review and meta-analysis. Clin Ther 2010;32(12):1987–2002.
45. Ludwin DB, Shafer SL. Con: the black box warning on droperidol should not be removed (but should be clarified!). Anesth Analg 2008;106(5):1418–20.
46. Habib AS, Gan TJ. Pro: the food and drug administration black box warning on droperidol is not justified. Anesth Analg 2008;106(5):1414–7.
47. Habib AS, Gan TJ. The use of droperidol before and after the Food and Drug Administration black box warning: a survey of the members of the society of ambulatory anesthesia. J Clin Anesth 2008;20(1):35–9.
48. FDA. 07/27/2009 [cited 2012 5th July]. Available at: http://www.fda.gov/safety/medwatch/safetyinformation/safetyalertsforhumanmedicalproducts/ucm173778. Accessed July 5, 2012.
49. George E, Hornuss C, Apfel CC. Neurokinin-1 and novel serotonin antagonists for postoperative and postdischarge nausea and vomiting. Curr Opin Anaesthesiol 2010;23(6):714–21.
50. Merker M, Kranke P, Morin AM, et al. Prophylaxis of nausea and vomiting in the postoperative phase: relative effectiveness of droperidol and metoclopramide. Anaesthesist 2011;60(5):432–40, 442–5. [in German].
51. Henzi I, Walder B, Tramer MR. Metoclopramide in the prevention of postoperative nausea and vomiting: a quantitative systematic review of randomized, placebo-controlled studies. Br J Anaesth 1999;83(5):761–71.
52. Schaub I, Lysakowski C, Elia N, et al. Low-dose droperidol (</=1 mg or </=15 mug kg-1) for the prevention of postoperative nausea and vomiting in adults: quantitative systematic review of randomised controlled trials. Eur J Anaesthesiol 2012;29(6):286–94.
53. Wallenborn J, Gelbrich G, Bulst D, et al. Prevention of postoperative nausea and vomiting by metoclopramide combined with dexamethasone: randomised double blind multicentre trial. BMJ 2006;333(7563):324.
54. Kranke P, Eberhart L. Übelkeit und Erbrechen in der perioperativen Phase (PONV). Köln (Germany): Deutscher Ärzte-Verlag; 2012.
55. Habib AS, Gan TJ. The effectiveness of rescue antiemetics after failure of prophylaxis with ondansetron or droperidol: a preliminary report. J Clin Anesth 2005; 17(1):62–5.
56. Gan TJ, Meyer TA, Apfel CC, et al. Society for Ambulatory Anesthesia guidelines for the management of postoperative nausea and vomiting. Anesth Analg 2007; 105(6):1615–28.
57. Kovac AL, O'Connor TA, Pearman MH, et al. Efficacy of repeat intravenous dosing of ondansetron in controlling postoperative nausea and vomiting: a randomized, double-blind, placebo-controlled multicenter trial. J Clin Anesth 1999;11(6):453–9.
58. DeBalli P. The use of propofol as an antiemetic. Int Anesthesiol Clin 2003;41(4): 67–77.
59. Gan TJ, El-Molem H, Ray J, et al. Patient-controlled antiemesis: a randomized, double-blind comparison of two doses of propofol versus placebo. Anesthesiology 1999;90(6):1564–70.
60. Borgeat A, Wilder-Smith OH, Wilder-Smith CH, et al. Adjuvant propofol for refractory cisplatin-associated nausea and vomiting. Lancet 1992;340(8820): 679–80.

61. Lee A, Fan LT. Stimulation of the wrist acupuncture point P6 for preventing postoperative nausea and vomiting. Cochrane Database Syst Rev 2009;(2). CD003281.

62. Pellegrini J, DeLoge J, Bennett J, et al. Comparison of inhalation of isopropyl alcohol vs promethazine in the treatment of postoperative nausea and vomiting (PONV) in patients identified as at high risk for developing PONV. AANA J 2009;77(4):293–9.

63. Cotton JW, Rowell LR, Hood RR, et al. A comparative analysis of isopropyl alcohol and ondansetron in the treatment of postoperative nausea and vomiting from the hospital setting to the home. AANA J 2007;75(1):21–6.

64. Teran L, Hawkins JK. The effectiveness of inhalation isopropyl alcohol vs. granisetron for the prevention of postoperative nausea and vomiting. AANA J 2007; 75(6):417–22.

65. Radford KD, Fuller TN, Bushey B, et al. Prophylactic isopropyl alcohol inhalation and intravenous ondansetron versus ondansetron alone in the prevention of postoperative nausea and vomiting in high-risk patients. AANA J 2011;79(Suppl 4): S69–74.

Postoperative Noninvasive Ventilation

Patrick J. Neligan, MD

KEYWORDS

- Postanesthesia care unit • Noninvasive ventilation
- Noninvasive positive pressure ventilation • Bilevel positive airway pressure
- Continuous positive airway pressure • Boussignac

KEY POINTS

- General anesthesia and surgery are associated with changes in the shape of the chest that result in atelectasis, a major factor in the development of postoperative respiratory failure.
- Postoperative noninvasive positive pressure ventilation (NIPPV) has been shown to improve oxygenation and ventilation for high-risk patients.
- NIPPV has been used as rescue therapy for patients developing acute respiratory distress postoperatively, and appears to be most frequently successful in patients whose problem is atelectasis or obesity.
- The use of continuous positive airway pressure (CPAP) helmets may improve patient comfort and compliance, and may result in fewer reintubations.
- Prophylactic NIPPV is usually preplanned. Rescue NIPPV is used in situations of central respiratory depression (pressure support ventilation), or for airway obstruction or low lung volumes (V/Q mismatch) (CPAP). Failure to respond to NIPPV after 20 minutes is usually an indication of intubation, mechanical ventilation, and transfer to the intensive care unit.

INTRODUCTION

General anesthesia is associated with significant changes in the shape of the chest, the orientation of the diaphragm, and alveolar gas content. This process results in significant loss of lung volume, airway closure, mucus trapping, ventilation-perfusion mismatch, and shunt, further compounded by surgeries of the upper abdomen and chest.[1] The major impact of these changes is atelectasis and increased work of breathing, which elevates the risk for reintubation, mechanical ventilation, and nosocomial pneumonia, all resulting in prolonged hospital stay.

The author has no conflicts of interest to disclose.
Department of Anesthesia & Intensive Care, Galway University Hospitals, Newcastle Road, Galway, Ireland
E-mail address: patrick.neligan@hse.ie

Anesthesiology Clin 30 (2012) 495–511
http://dx.doi.org/10.1016/j.anclin.2012.07.002　　　**anesthesiology.theclinics.com**

Noninvasive positive pressure ventilation (NIPPV **Box 1**), a term that covers continuous positive airway pressure (CPAP) and noninvasive pressure support ventilation (NIV/bilevel positive airway pressure [BiPAP]), is widely used in the postanesthesia care unit (PACU), intensive care unit (ICU), and high-dependency care unit (HDU) to both treat and prevent postoperative respiratory failure. This review initially addresses the basic physiology of gas-exchange abnormalities under anesthesia, and looks at NIPPV delivery systems and the evidence to support their use in the postoperative setting. Finally, a stepwise clinical approach to the patient with acute respiratory distress in the PACU is discussed.

GAS-EXCHANGE ABNORMALITIES UNDER ANESTHESIA
Anesthesia: Atelectasis and Ventilation-Perfusion Mismatch

Ventilation-perfusion mismatch occurs in all patients who undergo general anesthesia and major surgery,[2] and occurs whether or not the patient breathes spontaneously or whether the patient is maintained on volatile or intravenous anesthetic.[3] Immediately following induction of anesthesia there is a 16% to 20% reduction in functional residual capacity (FRC),[4] and this continues to decrease over the next 5 or 10 minutes.[5,6] The reduction in FRC is correlated with age and chest-wall elastance,[7] and leads to airway closure, reduced compliance, and ventilation-perfusion mismatch. The shape of the chest cavity changes: there is cephalad displacement of the diaphragm.[8] Complete or partial collapse of lung segments is known as atelectasis. Atelectasis occurs in 90% of anesthetized patients,[9] and is the most common cause of shunt (**Fig. 1**A). Up to 20% of lung bases are collapsed soon after induction of anesthesia.[6] Certain types of patients, namely the elderly and the obese, are at elevated risk for profound atelectasis, and certain types of surgery enhance risk: upper abdominal surgery, cardiac surgery, and thoracic surgery.

Oxygen and Atelectasis

Preoxygenation is known to increase the safe duration between apnea and hypoxemia; it involves breathing a high fractional inspired oxygen tension (Fio_2).[10,11] The vital capacity becomes a reservoir for apneic oxygenation, and depending on the shape and size of the patient there may be between 2 and 10 minutes of apnea-hypoxemia safety time.[12] However, this high Fio_2 causes atelectasis (absorption atelectasis; **Fig. 2**).[13] Atelectasis results from the presence of a large oxygen gradient between the alveolus and mixed venous blood: nitrogen washout removes the normal

---

Box 1
Delivery systems for noninvasive ventilation in the PACU

CPAP

CPAP face mask with positive end-expiratory pressure valve and high-flow system

Home BiPAP machine

Stand-alone noninvasive ventilator (such as BiPAP Vision)

Boussignac CPAP system

NIV

Home BiPAP machine

Stand-alone noninvasive ventilator (such as BiPAP Vision)

Intensive-care ventilator on "NIV" setting

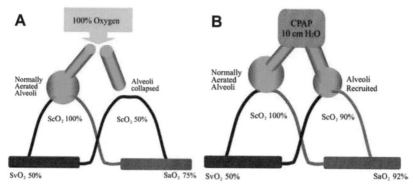

Fig. 1. (*A*) Impact of atelectasis on gas exchange. (*B*) Continuous positive airway pressure (CPAP) both recruits and prevents expiratory collapse of lung tissue, thus improving oxygenation. SaO_2, arterial oxygen saturation; ScO_2, oxyhemoglobin saturation of capillary blood; SvO_2, mixed venous oxygen saturation.

buttress for alveolar stability. Oxygen flows rapidly along the concentration gradient, and alveoli destabilize and collapse. Atelectasis also results from compression of pulmonary tissue (compression atelectasis), particularly the left lower lobe (compressed by the heart)[14] and the juxta-diaphragmatic region.[15] Although avoidance of preoxygenation prevents formation of atelectasis following induction of anesthesia,[16] the apneic safety margin is also lost.

Postoperative Hypoxemia

The major problem associated with intraoperative atelectasis is postoperative hypoxemia. On arrival at the recovery room (PACU), 20% of patients had an oxygen saturation of less than 92% and 10% had a saturation of less than 90% (if not transported on supplemental oxygen).[17] In patients undergoing upper abdominal surgery, the incidence of hypoxemia (pulse oximeter oxygen saturation [Spo_2] 86%–90%) was 38% and severe hypoxemia (Spo_2 85% or lower) was 3%. In patients undergoing thoracoabdominal surgery, the incidence of hypoxemia and severe hypoxemia were 52% and 20%, respectively.[18]

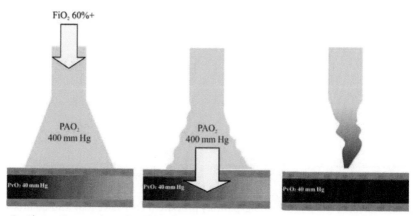

Fig. 2. Absorption atelectasis. FiO_2, fractional inspired oxygen tension; PAO_2, alveolar oxygen tension; PvO_2, mixed venous oxygen tension.

Postoperative atelectasis with associated hypoxemia and increased pulmonary workload is a problem for morbidly obese patients. Morbid obesity is associated with dramatic reductions in total respiratory system compliance.[19] Morbidly obese patients have significantly more atelectasis than nonobese patients, before induction (2.1% of total lung area vs 1.0%, P<.01), after tracheal extubation (7.6% vs 2.8%, P<.05), and 24 hours following (9.7% vs 1.9%, P<.01) laparoscopic surgery.[20]

Vital capacity and FRC decrease following extubation. This relationship varies linearly with body mass index.[21] Atelectasis increases the workload of breathing. In the PACU, the combination of partial neuromuscular blockade, opioids, and segmental lung collapse may lead to acute respiratory distress requiring reintubation. Of additional concern is the progressive increase in atelectasis that occurs over the first 24 hours in bariatric patients. Atelectasis and hypoventilation secondary to opioids, leading to hypercapnia-induced somnolence, may lead to airway obstruction and respiratory arrest.

A variety of interventions have been used intraoperatively to reduce the risk of atelectasis. Such approaches include preinduction CPAP,[22–24] intraoperative positive end-expiratory pressure (PEEP) with or without recruitment maneuvers,[25–27] and head-up or reverse-Trendelenburg patient positioning.[28–31] Despite these interventions, it has been found that 1 hour following admission to the PACU, patients had a significant loss of spirometric lung volume, suggesting that significant atelectasis occurs immediately following extubation.[32]

NONINVASIVE POSITIVE PRESSURE VENTILATION IN THE PACU

Noninvasive positive pressure ventilation (NIPPV) includes CPAP and pressure support ventilation/BiPAP, henceforth described as noninvasive ventilation (NIV). CPAP refers to elevated baseline airway pressure, applied throughout the respiratory cycle, but delivered principally at end expiration. It has 3 effects. (1) By restricting outward movement of gas from the alveoli, lung units are stented open, preventing end-expiratory atelectasis (**Fig. 1**B). (2) By increasing the gradient between the negative pleural pressure and the pressure at the airway, there is a decrease in the work of breathing for patients with a weak thoracic pump; this has the effect of recruiting collapsed lung units. (3) Positive pressure at the level of the upper airway stents opens distal airways and prevents dynamic airway collapse in expiration (gas trapping), and upper airway obstruction during inspiration and expiration. CPAP can be delivered through a tight-fitting full-face or nasal mask or helmet, attached to a PEEP valve (either adjustable or not) and a high-flow generating device (**Fig. 3**), or a noninvasive

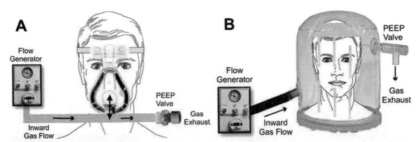

Fig. 3. (*A*) CPAP delivered through a face mask. In this illustration CPAP is delivered through a T-piece. However, the positive end-expiratory pressure (PEEP) valve may also be attached to the face mask. (*B*) CPAP delivered through a helmet. This helmet may also be used for noninvasive ventilation.

ventilator (see **Box 1**). CPAP can also be delivered by a proprietary mask-valve system known as Boussignac (Vygon, Montgomeryville, PA) using only an oxygen source; this device uses the Bernoulli principle, rather like a jet engine.[33]

The major complications of CPAP are patient intolerance and distress, lung hyperexpansion resulting in increased alveolar dead space and increased work of breathing, and increased intrathoracic pressure resulting in reduced venous return and hypotension.

Inspiratory pressure support may be added to CPAP: it is a patient-triggered, flow-cycled, pressure targeted mode of ventilation. Pressure support can be delivered through a modern anesthetic machine, an ICU-designated ventilator, or a stand-alone noninvasive ventilator (see **Box 1**). Pressure support reduces the workload of breathing by assisting the spontaneous breath in patients too weak to obtain normal tidal ventilation. The pressure support level is targeted at a tidal volume of 5 to 7 mL/kg body weight. When pressure support is delivered noninvasively from an ICU ventilator the plateau pressure (Pplat) is the pressure support plus the PEEP/CPAP level. Hence a patient receiving pressure support of 10 cm H_2O and PEEP of 5 cm H_2O has a Pplat of 15 cm H_2O. On a typical proprietary noninvasive ventilator, such as the BiPAP Vision (Philips Respironics, Andover, MD), different levels of airway pressure may be applied on inspiration (IPaP) and expiration (EPaP): in this scenario the plateau pressure is the IPaP level above atmospheric. For example, a patient receiving 10 cm H_2O IPaP and 5 cm H_2O EPaP has a Pplat of 10 cm H_2O.

Stand-alone noninvasive ventilators have several advantages for use in the PACU. Such ventilators have superior leak correction compared with ICU-type ventilators, such that, in the presence of a nasogastric tube or an ill-fitting mask, the device is capable of delivering the set airway pressure. Compared with basic NIV machines designed for use with obstructive sleep apnea (OSA) or chronic obstructive pulmonary disease, they are capable of delivering high inspired O_2 and, if necessary, mandatory ventilation. Compared with CPAP masks, these devices accurately measure respiratory rate and tidal ventilation and have apnea alarms. The disadvantage of these devices is cost and expertise: they are expensive devices that should only be used by trained practitioners.

NIV can be delivered by a face mask (**Fig. 4**), a nasal mask, or a helmet (see **Fig. 3B**). The latter is widely used in Europe, and is believed to be associated with greater

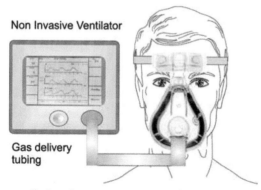

Fig. 4. Noninvasive ventilation. Pressure support ventilation is delivered through a stand-alone noninvasive ventilator. Gas flow is delivered via a single tubing system with powerful inspiratory and expiratory flow sensors. Different levels of PEEP and pressure support can be applied. In addition, a graphical waveform display gives the operator information about airway pressure, tidal volume, respiratory rate, and patient-ventilator synchrony.

patient comfort.[34] However, in the PACU the presence of a helmet may make communication problematic in patients requiring pain medications, and may elevate the risk associated with postoperative nausea and vomiting.

CLINICAL USE OF NIV IN THE PACU

NIV has been widely used in the recovery room in various settings, both prophylactic and therapeutic (**Box 2**). Although there have been several clinical studies that have evaluated postoperative NIPPV, most of these are small studies, few are randomized, and the majority look only at short-term outcomes. The literature can be neatly divided into studies that have addressed prophylactic NIPPV for patients who are at elevated risk for pulmonary complications, and rescue NIPPV for patients with postoperative respiratory distress. Studies have also evaluated continuous NIPPV following extubation or intermittent NIPPV for an hour or two each day for 2 or 3 days postoperatively.

PREVENTION OF PULMONARY COMPLICATIONS (PROPHYLACTIC NIV)

Patients who undergo upper abdominal, cardiac, thoracic, and bariatric surgery are at elevated risk for postoperative respiratory failure. For these patients prevention and reversal of atelectasis using NIPPV is an attractive proposition. Several studies have addressed this issue.

Prophylaxis After Cardiac Surgery

Patients who undergo cardiac surgery are known to have radiologically detectable atelectasis in the postoperative period. Several investigators have looked at NIV in this setting. Thirty patients who underwent coronary artery bypass grafting (CABG)

Box 2
Indications for NIPPV in the PACU

Prophylactic

1. Prevention of airway obstruction
    a. Obstructive sleep apnea-hypopnea syndrome
    b. Tracheomalacia following thyroidectomy
2. Prevention of atelectasis in high-risk surgical patients such as those who have undergone bariatric surgery

Therapeutic

3. Treatment of postoperative hypoxemia
    a. Atelectasis
    b. Mucus plugging
4. Treatment of postoperative hypercarbia or respiratory weakness
    a. Residual neuromuscular blockade
    b. Diaphragmatic weakness
    c. Delayed emergence from anesthesia
    d. Phrenic nerve paralysis (eg, following interscalene block)
    e. High neuraxial block
5. Treatment of postobstructive pulmonary edema

were randomized to receive oxygen-therapy CPAP for 8 hours after extubation.[35] Oxygenation was significantly better in the CPAP group at the end of this period. However, by the second postoperative morning oxygenation was equally poor in both groups, inferring that early postoperative CPAP failed to prevent late atelectasis.

Thomas and colleagues[36] demonstrated that CPAP for 1 hour after CABG surgery reduced the shunt fraction and reduced the subjective workload of breathing. Matte and colleagues[37] demonstrated that both CPAP and NIV improved oxygenation and lung volumes in patients after CABG during the first 2 postoperative days. Pinilla and colleagues[38] randomized postoperative cardiac surgery patients to nasal CPAP (nCPAP), for 12 hours, or oxygen following extubation. Although oxygenation was better for the first 24 hours in the nCPAP group, this benefit did not persist subsequently.

Is intermittent NIPPV effective? One-hundred fifty patients following cardiac surgery were randomized to CPAP (5 cm H_2O) or NIV 4 times a day for 30 minutes.[39] NIV (pressure support) was associated with reduced atelectasis on chest radiography, but there was no difference in oxygenation pulmonary function tests or length of stay between the groups. Hence, NIV is not superior to CPAP in the prevention of postoperative lung dysfunction in this setting.[40] Zarbock and colleagues[41] randomized 500 patients who underwent cardiac surgery to intermittent nasal nCPAP at 10 cm H_2O for 10 minutes every 4 hours (controls) or continuous CPAP at 10 cm H_2O for at least 6 hours. Prophylactic continuous nCPAP (PCnCPAP) significantly improved arterial oxygenation (partial pressure of arterial oxygen [Pao_2]/Fio_2 [PF] ratio) without adverse hemodynamic consequences. Pulmonary complications including hypoxemia (defined as PF ratio <100), pneumonia, and reintubation rate were reduced in PCnCPAP patients compared with controls (12 of 232 patients vs 25 of 236 patients, respectively; P = .03). The readmission rate to the ICU or HDU was significantly lower in PCnCPAP patients (7 of 232 patients vs 14 of 236 patients, respectively; P = .03). This study demonstrates that if CPAP is to be effective, it must be given continuously for a sustained period postoperatively.

Prophylaxis After Thoracic Surgery

NIPPV has been used extensively following thoracic and thoracoabdominal surgery. Aguiló and colleagues[42] studied 19 patients who had undergone lung resection and randomized them to NIV (BiPAP) or oxygen for 1 hour postoperatively. In the study group, NIV increased Pao_2 and decreased alveolar to arterial oxygen pressure gradient. Of interest, improved oxygenation persisted in this group1 hour after withdrawing NIV and there were no complications associated with NIV. Similar data have been reported following bilateral lung transplantation.[43]

Seventy patients undergoing thoracoabdominal esophagectomy were randomized to postoperative inspiratory resistance–positive expiratory pressure (IR-PEP) or CPAP.[44] Significantly fewer patients in the CPAP group required reintubation (P<.05).

Kindgen-Milles and colleagues[45] studied 56 patients who underwent thoracoabdominal aortic aneurysm repair, randomized to CPAP for 12 to 24 hours following extubation or standard oxygen therapy. The application of CPAP was associated with fewer pulmonary complications compared with the control group (7 of 25 patients vs 24 of 25 subjects, P = .019). Patients in the CPAP group remained in hospital for fewer days (22 ± 2 vs 34 ± 5 days, P = .048) and had better oxygenation without hemodynamic complications.

Is preoperative NIV beneficial in the postoperative period? Few data are available. Perrin and colleagues[46] studied 32 patients scheduled for elective pulmonary lobectomy randomized to preoperative and postoperative (for 3 days) NIV versus standard treatment. NIV improved blood gases and spirometry both preoperatively and postoperatively through day 1 following surgery. Hospital stay was significantly longer in the control group than in the NIV group ($P = .04$).

Prophylactic NIV After General Surgery

Bagan and colleagues[47] randomized patients to NIV versus oxygen therapy following aortic surgery. The incidence of pulmonary complications (0/14 [0%] vs 5/15 [33%], $P = .004$) and hospital length of stay in intensive care was shorter in the NIV group (2.5 vs 6.5 days, $P<.001$). Böhner and colleagues[48] prospectively studied 204 patients who underwent midline laparotomy for vascular surgery. The patients were randomized to receive nCPAP or standard therapy during the first postoperative night. nCPAP significantly reduced the number of patients with severe hypoxemia, defined as PF ratio less than 1.0 (5 vs 17, $P = .01$). Despite this, there were no other outcome differences.

Regarding NIV following abdominal surgery, Stock and colleagues[49] intermittently administered CPAP in patients after upper abdominal surgery. Compared with standard therapy (incentive spirometry or coughing and deep breathing), the CPAP group recovered their FRC more quickly and had significantly less atelectasis on chest radiography at 72 hours. Denehy and colleagues[50] undertook a similar study in which intermittent CPAP was administered intermittently 4 times a day, in addition to physiotherapy, to postoperative patients versus no NIV. There were no significant differences in outcomes. Ricksten and colleagues[51] demonstrated that intermittent CPAP over 3 days reduced atelectasis compared with controls; the clinical significance of this is unclear. Again, it is likely that continuous NIPPV is superior to intermittent therapy in this patient subgroup.

However, patient selection is clearly important. Carlsson and colleagues[52] randomized 24 patients who had undergone elective cholecystectomy to CPAP for 4 h after surgery or oxygen therapy. Although both groups had a reduction in vital capacity and Pao_2 and chest-radiographic evidence of atelectasis, there were no differences in outcomes.

Prophylactic NIV After Bariatric Surgery

There has been a dramatic increase in the number of bariatric surgical procedures performed worldwide over the past 2 decades. Although major complications of these surgeries are relatively rare, patients are at risk for postoperative respiratory failure, and several investigators have looked at NIV in this setting. Ebeo and colleagues[53] evaluated the effect of NIV (BiPAP) on pulmonary function in obese patients following open gastric bypass surgery. Of the 27 patients recruited, 14 received NIV and 13 received conventional postoperative care. Forced vital capacity and forced expiratory volume in 1 second were significantly higher on each of the 3 consecutive postoperative days in the patients who received NIV. The Spo_2 was significantly decreased in the control group over the same time period. These improved measures of pulmonary function, however, did not translate into fewer hospital days or lower complication rates.

Joris and colleagues[54] studied 30 patients who had undergone bariatric surgery, assigned to either no NIPPV, low levels of NIV (8/4 cm H_2O), or higher levels of NIV (12/4 cm H_2O). Spirometry was performed the day before surgery, 24 hours after surgery, and on days 2 and 3. Oxygen saturation by pulse oximeter (Spo_2) was also recorded during room air breathing. The patients receiving the higher NIV settings had significantly better spirometry and Spo_2 24 hours following surgery, and this benefit was evident over the following 2 days. Another study of NIV following

Roux-en-Y gastric bypass[55] showed that patients who received NIV had better spirometry and oxygenation on the first postoperative day.

Gaszynski and colleagues[56] randomized 19 patients who underwent gastric bypass surgery to Boussignac CPAP or oxygen therapy. The CPAP group had significantly better oxygenation postoperatively, with no difference in $Paco_2$.

Postoperative NIV therefore appears to improve oxygenation in morbidly obese patients who undergo bariatric surgery. Regarding other surgeries in the same subpopulation, Zoremba and colleagues[57] randomized 60 obese patients undergoing extremity surgery (body mass index 30–45 kg/m^2) to NIV in the PACU or oxygen therapy. Patients given NIV had significantly better spirometry values and oxygenation on discharge to the ward, and this persisted for 24 hours.

When is the correct timing of administration of postoperative NIPPV? Neligan and colleagues[32] evaluated 40 patients who underwent bariatric surgery and received preinduction CPAP, intraoperative PEEP, and recruitment maneuvers. One group were administered CPAP via the Boussignac system immediately following extubation (and in the recovery room); the other group were transported to the recovery room where, after 30 minutes, they received CPAP. Immediate postextubation CPAP resulted in dramatic improvements in spirometric lung function that, again, persisted for 24 hours. Thus there is a significant loss of lung volume in bariatric patients following extubation, and much of this can be prevented if CPAP is applied immediately.

THERAPEUTIC NIPPV IN PATIENTS WITH POSTOPERATIVE RESPIRATORY FAILURE

In patients who develop acute postoperative respiratory failure in the PACU/ICU, NIPPV has the potential to reduce the length of stay in ICU and development of further complications by preventing reintubation.

Respiratory failure following thoracic surgery is associated with very poor outcomes. Auriant and colleagues[58] compared NIV versus medical therapy for respiratory failure following lung resection. Five of the 24 patients (20.8%) randomly assigned to the NIPPV group versus 12 of the 24 patients (50%) assigned to the no-NIPPV group required intubation ($P = .035$). Three (12.5%) patients in the NIPPV group died versus 9 (37.5%) patients in the no-NIPPV group ($P = .045$). A prospective observational study[59] conducted over 4 years on similar patients showed that NIV was successful in this setting in 85.3% of cases. In patients who failed NIV the mortality rate was 46%; the major risk factors for failure were cardiac morbidities and failure to respond initially. Hence, failure of NIV following lung resection predicts adverse outcomes.

Michelet and colleagues[60] performed a case-control study of patients who either received NIV or oxygen therapy for respiratory failure following esophagectomy. NIV was associated with a lower reintubation rate (9 vs 23 patients; $P = .008$), lower frequency of acute respiratory distress syndrome (ARDS) (8 vs 19 patients; $P = .015$), and a shortened ICU stay (mean 14 vs 22 days; $P = .034$). NIV patients had a substantially lower incidence of anastomotic dehiscence (2 vs 10; $P = .027$). This finding suggests that there may have been a selection bias in the dataset, as NIV is unlikely to prevent wound complications; anastomotic dehiscence is more likely to cause persistent inflammation, sepsis, and lung injury.

García-Delgado and colleagues[61] retrospectively evaluated 1225 postcardiac surgical patients, 63 (5.1%) of whom underwent NIV for respiratory failure after extubation. There was a significant delay between extubation and NIV, a median time of 40 hours (range 18–96 hours). NIV failed in 52.4% of patients, and was associated with higher hospital mortality (51.5% vs 6.7%, $P = .001$) NIV failure was predicted by early respiratory distress (within 24 hours of extubation) and lower pH. Atelectasis and obesity were associated with better results from NIV.

Regarding abdominal surgery, In a cohort of 72 patients who had been readmitted to ICU with respiratory failure following such surgery, NIV successfully prevented reintubation in 67%.[62] Narita and colleagues[63] undertook a retrospective study of patients who did and did not receive NIV after liver resection whereby there was respiratory distress or significant atelectasis. Respiratory-cause mortality was significantly lower in the NIV group than in the non-NIV group (0.0% vs 40.0%, P = .007). There was no statistically significant difference in overall mortality. Oxygenation was significantly better after NIV treatment at 24 hours. The rate of reintubation was significantly lower in the NIV group (12.5% vs 50.0%, P = .04). Although these results seem impressive, this was a retrospective cohort study with a strong likelihood of systematic bias.

Antonelli and colleagues[64] randomized 40 patients who developed acute respiratory failure following solid organ transplantation to either NIV or oxygen therapy. The use of NIV was associated with improved oxygenation, a significant reduction in the rate of endotracheal intubation (20% vs 70%; P = .002), rate of fatal complications (20% vs 50%; P = .05), length of stay in the ICU by survivors (mean [SD] days, 5.5 [3] vs 9 [4]; P = .03), and ICU mortality (20% vs 50%; P = .05) Of importance, however, hospital mortality did not differ between the groups.

Does the delivery system make a difference? Redondo Calvo and colleagues[65] reported on outcomes over 2 years of patients treated with helmet CPAP/NIV in a surgical ICU. Ninety-nine patients were treated with the helmet, with a 75% success rate. The investigators reported 3 independent risk factors for failure of NIV: ARDS, pneumonia, and lack of improvement with NIV in 1 hour. Conti and colleagues[66] reported improved outcomes in patients with respiratory failure following abdominal surgery who received NIV through a helmet versus historical controls who had received a NIV via face mask. The helmet appeared to be better tolerated than the face mask, and there were fewer treatment failures in this group.

Squadrone and colleagues[67] studied 209 consecutive patients who had undergone elective major abdominal surgery and developed postoperative hypoxemia. The patients were randomized to receive either oxygen therapy or helmet CPAP in the recovery room. Patients who received oxygen plus CPAP had a lower reintubation rate (1% vs 10%; P = .005) and a lower occurrence of pneumonia (2% vs 10%, P = .02), infection (3% vs 10%, P = .03), and sepsis (2% vs 9%; P = .03) than did patients treated with oxygen alone. It should be noted that patients in this study received intramuscular opioids rather than epidural analgesia.

Keenan and colleagues[68] randomized 81 postoperative patients who developed respiratory distress within 48 hours of extubation to medical therapy or NIV. There was no difference in the rate of reintubation (72% vs 69%; relative risk, 1.04; 95% confidence interval, 0.78–1.38) or hospital mortality (31% for both groups; relative risk, 0.99; 95% confidence interval, 0.52–1.91). However, this should be considered a study of NIV in surgical critical care rather than in postoperative care. The patients had been intubated postoperatively for a mean of 3.4 and 5.0 days in the NIV and medical therapy groups, respectively. Patients had ARDS by blood gas criteria and very high APACHE II (Acute Physiology and Chronic Health Evaluation II) scores (in excess of 20). These data are consistent with evidence for ineffectiveness of NIV in ARDS and sepsis.[69]

CLINICAL APPROACH

The decision to use NIPPV in the PACU for prophylactic therapy in high-risk patients is usually taken preoperatively, based on sleep studies (for OSA) or on assessment of risk. There is no evidence that NIV is superior to CPAP in these situations. The applied airway pressure will depend on the patient's body habitus (higher body mass index will require greater amounts of positive pressure) and intraoperative oxygenation. For morbidly obese patients (body mass index >40 kg/m^2), CPAP of 10 cm H_2O is recommended.

The remainder of this discussion focuses on patients who develop acute respiratory distress in the PACU.

Acute Respiratory Distress

A variety of problems lead to acute respiratory distress in the PACU. The key to making the diagnosis is to look at the patient's breathing pattern. If the patient is taking rapid breaths (>30 breaths per minute) but with apparently normal tidal volumes, a nonpulmonary source should be considered: pain, anxiety, delirium, a full bladder, and so forth. If the patient is taking slow shallow breaths, with normal synchrony between opening of the mouth to inhale and movement of the chest outward and downward, the problem is most likely ventilatory failure secondary to central respiratory depression. This failure most commonly results from opioid administration, but may also follow the administration of midazolam/lorazepam or discontinuation of a propofol infusion.

If the patient is taking rapid shallow breaths, the problem is either ventilatory failure secondary to a peripheral problem or oxygenation failure secondary to ventilation-perfusion mismatch (**Fig. 5**). The key to separating the two is the clinical circumstance and the presence or absence of hypoxemia (low Spo_2 or requirement for high Fio_2). In the absence of hypoxemia, a neuromuscular problem should be considered, such as residual neuromuscular blockade or a dense epidural block that paralyzes the intercostal muscles. One also sees this pattern in patients with low physiologic reserve, the malnourished, and the critically ill. In patients who have undergone thoracic surgery or retroperitoneal surgery, a high clinical suspicion for pneumothorax should be considered; this is characterized by hypoxemia, unilateral breath sounds and, in severe cases, hypotension.

Rapid shallow breathing with hypoxemia is caused by ventilation-perfusion mismatch, usually caused by retained secretions and/or atelectasis. This condition most commonly occurs in patients who have undergone abdominal or thoracic surgery, are morbidly obese, or have been positioned intraoperatively in the Trendelenburg position.

Pulmonary embolism should be suspected in patients who have undergone pelvic or hip surgery and have rapid shallow breathing and hypoxemia, associated with tachycardia and hypotension.

An obstructed breathing pattern is suggestive of upper or middle airway abnormality. The problem is caused by central loss of pharyngeal tone, and soft-tissue obstruction (associated with depressed level of consciousness and anesthesia) or mechanical obstruction to the airway: above, at the level of, or below the glottis. Classically the patient has nasal flaring, supraclavicular or intercostal retraction, and a seesaw chest movement: the chest moves inwards as the diaphragm descends. The patient may have inspiratory stridor (supraglottic obstruction), expiratory stridor (glottic or subglottic obstruction), or expiratory wheeze (bronchospasm). Typically hypoxemia is a late complication of airway obstruction. This aspect is important, as hypoxia may be rapidly followed by bradycardia and asystole.

Treating the Problem

The patient should nursed in the upright or seated position: the effect of gravity is to recruit lung tissue and increase FRC. Oxygen should be administered and the patient

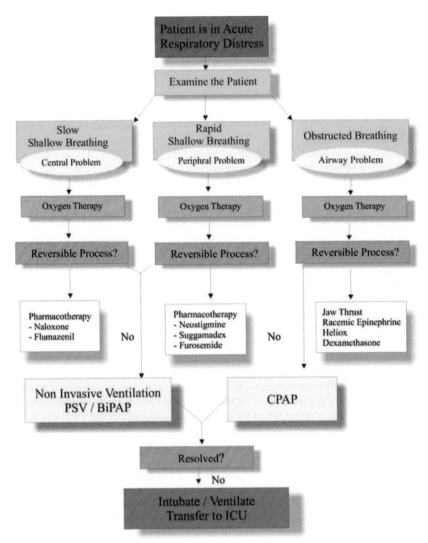

Fig. 5. Noninvasive positive pressure ventilation for acute postoperative respiratory distress. PSA, procedural sedation and analgesia.

should be encouraged to cough, to mobilize secretions, and take deep breaths. Attention should be given to potential reversibility of the process. If the patient is taking slow shallow breaths caused by opioids or benzodiazepines, consideration should be given to naloxone or flumazenil administration. If the patient has stridor, secondary to laryngeal edema, he or she may benefit from racemic epinephrine, steroids and, if available, heliox (helium and oxygen gas mixture). If the patient has rapid shallow breathing, partial neuromuscular blockade should be immediately considered, and reversal administered: neostigmine or sugammadex. If the patient previously demonstrated an obstructed breathing pattern and now has rapid shallow breathing, postobstructive pulmonary ("negative pressure") edema should be considered: furosemide 20 to 40 mg intravenously may improve symptoms. In each case, if immediate reversal of the problem is not possible, noninvasive ventilation should be considered. As a bridging exercise, the anesthesiologist may support the airway using a Mapleson-C circuit or similar device, with the APL (pressure release) valve partially closed down.

When commencing NIPPV, the mechanism of respiratory distress should be considered. NIPPV is suitable only for patients whose problem would be expected to resolve within 4 to 6 hours. Hence a hypoxemic distressed patient who has atelectasis is a good candidate for NIPPV; a patient who aspirated gastric contents, with a similar clinical picture, is not. Comatose or severely agitated patients and those on full stomachs (pregnant or emergency surgical patients) are not suitable for NIPPV. Nor are patients with copious oral or nasal secretions, or those that are bleeding from their mouths, lungs, or upper gastrointestinal tract.

Patients with rapid shallow breathing or obstructive breathing patterns are likely to respond to CPAP: this restores FRC, helps recruit the lung, and prevents dynamic airway collapse and air trapping. CPAP of 5 to 10 cm H_2O is usually sufficient; the level of support is titrated against the patient's respiratory rate and Spo_2. Excessive end-expiratory pressure increases dead space and increases the work of breathing. If the patient's oxygenation improves but respiratory rate remains high (>30/min), pressure support can be added.

Patients with slow shallow breathing tend to hypoventilate and retain CO_2: there is inadequate alveolar ventilation, and they are more likely to benefit from NIV. Pressure support is titrated against the patient's tidal volume: a target range of 5 to 7 mL/kg. Typical values are 5 to 10 cm H_2O above the PEEP level. With the exception of patients with severe bullous emphysematous lung disease, PEEP is always added because, irrespective of the mechanism of injury, all patients with postoperative respiratory distress are at risk for atelectasis.

In general, if patients respond to NIPPV then their symptoms settle down rapidly, usually within 15 minutes. If after 15 to 20 minutes the patient's respiratory rate continues to exceed 30 breaths per minute, if the Spo_2 is less than 90%, or if the patient becomes hypotensive or comatose, the patient should be intubated and transferred to the ICU.

SUMMARY

NIPPV is a useful tool that may be used for select patients in the PACU. NIPPV can be used to prevent and treat postoperative respiratory failure. This approach may reduce the number of patients being reintubated in the PACU as well as the burden on ICU beds, the length of stay in hospital, and morbidity.

REFERENCES

1. Arozullah AM, Daley J, Henderson WG, et al. Multifactorial risk index for predicting postoperative respiratory failure in men after major noncardiac surgery. The National Veterans Administration Surgical Quality Improvement Program. Ann Surg 2000;232:242–53.
2. Lundquist H, Hedenstierna G, Strandberg A, et al. CT-assessment of dependent lung densities in man during general anesthesia. Acta Radiol 1995;36:626–32.
3. Strandberg A, Tokics L, Hedenstierna G, et al. Constitutional factors promoting development of atelectasis during anesthesia. Acta Anaesthesiol Scand 1987; 31:21–4.
4. Hedenstierna G, Edmark L. The effects of anesthesia and muscle paralysis on the respiratory system. Intensive Care Med 2005;31:1327–35.

5. Magnusson L, Spahn DR. New concepts of atelectasis during general anesthesia. Br J Anaesth 2003;91:61–72.
6. Hedenstierna G. Alveolar collapse and closure of airways: regular effects of anesthesia. Clin Physiol Funct Imaging 2003;23:123–9.
7. Reber A, Engberg G, Hedenstierna G, et al. Volumetric analysis of aeration in the lungs during general anesthesia. Br J Anaesth 1996;76:760–6.
8. Reber A, Nylund U, Hedenstierna G. Position and shape of the diaphragm: implications for atelectasis formation. Anaesthesia 1998;53:1054–61.
9. Gunnarsson L, Tokics L, Gustavsson H, et al. Influence of age on atelectasis formation and gas exchange impairment during general anesthesia. Br J Anaesth 1991;66:423–32.
10. Pandit JJ, Duncan T, Robbins PA. Total oxygen uptake with two maximal breathing techniques and the tidal volume breathing technique: a physiologic study of preoxygenation. Anesthesiology 2003;99:841–6.
11. Drummond GB, Park GR. Arterial oxygen-saturation before intubation of the trachea an assessment of oxygenation techniques. Br J Anaesth 1984;56:987–93.
12. Gander S, Frascarolo P, Suter M, et al. Positive end-expiratory pressure during induction of general anesthesia increases duration of nonhypoxic apnea in morbidly obese patients. Anesth Analg 2005;100:580–4.
13. Rothen HU, Sporre B, Engberg G, et al. Reexpansion of atelectasis during general anesthesia may have a prolonged effect. Acta Anaesthesiol Scand 1995;39:118–25.
14. Malbouisson LM, Busch CJ, Puybasset L, et al. CT Scan ARDS Study Group: role of the heart in the loss of aeration characterizing lower lobes in acute respiratory distress syndrome. Am J Respir Crit Care Med 2000;161:2005–12.
15. Hedenstierna G. Atelectasis and its prevention during anesthesia. Eur J Anaesthesiol 1998;15:387–90.
16. Rothen HU, Sporre B, Engberg G, et al. Prevention of atelectasis during general anesthesia. Lancet 1995;345:1387–91.
17. Mathes DD, Conaway MR, Ross WT. Ambulatory surgery: room air versus nasal cannula oxygen during transport after general anesthesia. Anesth Analg 2001;93:917–21.
18. Xue FS, Li BW, Zhang GS, et al. The influence of surgical sites on early postoperative hypoxemia in adults undergoing elective surgery. Anesth Analg 1999;88:213–9.
19. Pelosi P, Croci M, Ravagnan I. The effects of body mass on lung volumes, respiratory mechanics, and gas exchange during general anesthesia. Anesth Analg 1998;87:654–60.
20. Eichenberger A, Proietti S, Wicky S, et al. Morbid obesity and postoperative pulmonary atelectasis: an underestimated problem. Anesth Analg 2002;95:1788–92.
21. Ungern-Sternberg BS, Regli A, Schneider MC, et al. Effect of obesity and site of surgery on perioperative lung volumes. Br J Anaesth 2004;92:202–7.
22. Rusca M, Proietti S, Schnyder P, et al. Prevention of atelectasis formation during induction of general anesthesia. Anesth Analg 2003;97:1835–9.
23. Herriger A, Frascarolo P, Magnusson L. The effect of positive airway pressure during pre-oxygenation and induction of anesthesia upon duration of nonhypoxic apnoea. Anaesthesia 2004;59:243–7.
24. Coussa M, Proietti S, Schnyder P, et al. Prevention of atelectasis formation during the induction of general anesthesia in morbidly obese patients. Anesth Analg 2004;98:1491–5, table.

25. Rothen HU, Sporre B, Engberg G, et al. Re-expansion of atelectasis during general anesthesia: a computed tomography study. Br J Anaesth 1993;71:788–95.

26. Rothen HU, Neumann P, Berglund JE, et al. Dynamics of re-expansion of atelectasis during general anesthesia. Br J Anaesth 1999;82:551–6.

27. Yoshino J, Akata T, Takahashi S. Intraoperative changes in arterial oxygenation during volume-controlled mechanical ventilation in modestly obese patients undergoing laparotomies with general anesthesia. Acta Anaesthesiol Scand 2003;47:742–50.

28. Lane S, Saunders D, Schofield A, et al. A prospective, randomised controlled trial comparing the efficacy of pre-oxygenation in the 20 degrees head-up vs supine position. Anaesthesia 2005;60:1064–7.

29. Dixon BJ, Dixon JB, Carden JR, et al. Preoxygenation is more effective in the 25 degrees head-up position than in the supine position in severely obese patients: a randomized controlled study. Anesthesiology 2005;102:1110–5.

30. Baraka AS, Hanna MT, Jabbour SI, et al. Preoxygenation of pregnant and nonpregnant women in the head-up versus supine position. Anesth Analg 1992;75:757–9.

31. Perilli V, Sollazzi L, Modesti C, et al. Comparison of positive end-expiratory pressure with reverse Trendelenburg position in morbidly obese patients undergoing bariatric surgery: effects on hemodynamics and pulmonary gas exchange. Obes Surg 2003;13:605–9.

32. Neligan PJ, Malhotra G, Ochroch EA, et al. Continuous positive airway pressure via the Boussignac system immediately after extubation improves lung function in morbidly obese patients with obstructive sleep apnea undergoing laparoscopic bariatric surgery. Anesthesiology 2009;110:878–84.

33. Moritz F, Benichou J, Vanheste M, et al. Boussignac continuous positive airway pressure device in the emergency care of acute cardiogenic pulmonary oedema: a randomized pilot study. Eur J Emerg Med 2003;10:204–8.

34. Chiumello D, Pelosi P, Gattinoni L, et al. Noninvasive positive pressure ventilation delivered by helmet vs. standard face mask. Intensive Care Med 2003;29:1671–9.

35. Jousela I, Rasanen J, Verkkala K, et al. Continuous positive airway pressure by mask in patients after coronary surgery. Acta Anaesthesiol Scand 1994;38:311–6.

36. Thomas AN, Ryan JP, Doran BR. Nasal CPAP after coronary artery surgery. Anaesthesia 1992;47:316–9.

37. Matte P, Jacquet L, Van DM, et al. Effects of conventional physiotherapy, continuous positive airway pressure and non-invasive ventilatory support with bilevel positive airway pressure after coronary artery bypass grafting. Acta Anaesthesiol Scand 2000;44:75–81.

38. Pinilla JC, Oleniuk FH, Tan L, et al. Use of a nasal continuous positive airway pressure mask in the treatment of postoperative atelectasis in aortocoronary bypass surgery. Crit Care Med 1990;18:836–40.

39. Pasquina P, Merlani P, Granier JM. Continuous positive airway pressure versus noninvasive pressure support ventilation to treat atelectasis after cardiac surgery. Anesth Analg 2004;99:1001–8, table.

40. Liao G, Chen R, He J. Prophylactic use of noninvasive positive pressure ventilation in post-thoracic surgery patients: a prospective randomized control study. J Thorac Dis 2010;2:205–9.

41. Zarbock A, Mueller E, Kindgen-Milles D, et al. Prophylactic nasal continuous positive airway pressure following cardiac surgery protects from postoperative pulmonary complications: a prospective, randomized, controlled trial in 500 patients. Chest 2009;135:1252–9.

42. Aguiló R, Togores B, Pons S, et al. Noninvasive ventilatory support after lung resectional surgery. Chest 1997;112:117–21.
43. Rocco M, Conti G, Antonelli M, et al. Non-invasive pressure support ventilation in patients with acute respiratory failure after bilateral lung transplantation. Intensive Care Med 2001;27:1622–6.
44. Fagevik OM, Wennberg E, Johnsson E. Randomized clinical study of the prevention of pulmonary complications after thoracoabdominal resection by two different breathing techniques. Br J Surg 2002;89:1228–34.
45. Kindgen-Milles D, Muller E, Buhl R, et al. Nasal-continuous positive airway pressure reduces pulmonary morbidity and length of hospital stay following thoracoabdominal aortic surgery. Chest 2005;128:821–8.
46. Perrin C, Jullien V, Venissac N, et al. Prophylactic use of noninvasive ventilation in patients undergoing lung resectional surgery. Respir Med 2007;101:1572–8.
47. Bagan P, Bouayad M, Benabdesselam A. Prevention of pulmonary complications after aortic surgery: evaluation of prophylactic noninvasive perioperative ventilation. Ann Vasc Surg 2011;25:920–2.
48. Böhner H, Kindgen-Milles D, Grust A. Prophylactic nasal continuous positive airway pressure after major vascular surgery: results of a prospective randomized trial. Langenbecks Arch Surg 2002;387:21–6.
49. Stock MC, Downs JB, Gauer PK. Prevention of postoperative pulmonary complications with CPAP, incentive spirometry, and conservative therapy. Chest 1985;87:151–7.
50. Denehy L, Carroll S, Ntoumenopoulos G. A randomized controlled trial comparing periodic mask CPAP with physiotherapy after abdominal surgery. Physiother Res Int 2001;6:236–50.
51. Ricksten SE, Bengtsson A, Soderberg C. Effects of periodic positive airway pressure by mask on postoperative pulmonary function. Chest 1986;89:774–81.
52. Carlsson C, Sonden B, Thylen U. Can postoperative continuous positive airway pressure (CPAP) prevent pulmonary complications after abdominal surgery? Intensive Care Med 1981;7:225–9.
53. Ebeo CT, Benotti PN, Byrd RP Jr. The effect of bi-level positive airway pressure on postoperative pulmonary function following gastric surgery for obesity. Respir Med 2002;96:672–6.
54. Joris JL, Sottiaux TM, Chiche JD. Effect of bi-level positive airway pressure (Bi-PAP) nasal ventilation on the postoperative pulmonary restrictive syndrome in obese patients undergoing gastroplasty. Chest 1997;111:665–70.
55. Pessoa KC, Araujo GF, Pinheiro AN. Noninvasive ventilation in the immediate postoperative of gastrojejunal derivation with Roux-en-Y gastric bypass. Rev Bras Fisioter 2010;14:290–5 [Article in English, Portuguese].
56. Gaszynski T, Tokarz A, Piotrowski D, et al. Boussignac CPAP in the postoperative period in morbidly obese patients. Obes Surg 2007;17:452–6.
57. Zoremba M, Kalmus G, Begemann D, et al. Short term non-invasive ventilation post-surgery improves arterial blood-gases in obese subjects compared to supplemental oxygen delivery—a randomized controlled trial. BMC Anesthesiol 2011;11:10.
58. Auriant I, Jallot A, Herve P, et al. Noninvasive ventilation reduces mortality in acute respiratory failure following lung resection. Am J Respir Crit Care Med 2001;164:1231–5.
59. Lefebvre A, Lorut C, Alifano M, et al. Noninvasive ventilation for acute respiratory failure after lung resection: an observational study. Intensive Care Med 2009;35:663–70.

60. Michelet P, D'Journo XB, Seinaye F, et al. Non-invasive ventilation for treatment of postoperative respiratory failure after oesophagectomy. Br J Surg 2009;96:54–60.
61. García-Delgado M, Navarrete I, García-Palma MJ, et al. Postoperative respiratory failure after cardiac surgery: use of noninvasive ventilation. J Cardiothorac Vasc Anesth 2012;26:443–7.
62. Jaber S, Delay JM, Chanques G, et al. Outcomes of patients with acute respiratory failure after abdominal surgery treated with noninvasive positive pressure ventilation. Chest 2005;128:2688–95.
63. Narita M, Tanizawa K, Chin K, et al. Noninvasive ventilation improves the outcome of pulmonary complications after liver resection. Intern Med 2010;49:1501–7.
64. Antonelli M, Conti G, Bufi M, et al. Noninvasive ventilation for treatment of acute respiratory failure in patients undergoing solid organ transplantation: a randomized trial. JAMA 2000;283:235–41.
65. Redondo Calvo FJ, Madrazo M, Gilsanz F, et al. Helmet noninvasive mechanical ventilation in patients with acute postoperative respiratory failure. Respir Care 2012;57:743–52.
66. Conti G, Cavaliere F, Costa R, et al. Noninvasive positive-pressure ventilation with different interfaces in patients with respiratory failure after abdominal surgery: a matched-control study. Respir Care 2007;52:1463–71.
67. Squadrone V, Coha M, Ranieri VM, et al. Continuous positive airway pressure for treatment of postoperative hypoxemia: a randomized controlled trial. JAMA 2005; 293:589–95.
68. Keenan SP, Powers C, McCormack DG, et al. Noninvasive positive-pressure ventilation for postextubation respiratory distress: a randomized controlled trial. JAMA 2002;287:3238–44.
69. Agarwal R, Aggarwal AN, Gupta D. Role of noninvasive ventilation in acute lung injury/acute respiratory distress syndrome: a proportion meta-analysis. Respir Care 2010;55:1653–60.

Decreased Urine Output and Acute Kidney Injury in the Postanesthesia Care Unit

Kara Beth Chenitz, MD[a,1], Meghan B. Lane-Fall, MD[b,1,*]

KEYWORDS

- Acute kidney injury • Acute renal failure • Postanesthesia care
- Postoperative oliguria

KEY POINTS

- Decreased urine output is a common occurrence in the postanesthesia care unit (PACU).
- Acute kidney injury (AKI) is uncommon in the PACU, but it is associated with increased morbidity and mortality.
- Maintaining adequate renal perfusion by ensuring euvolemia and normotension is key to preventing the development of AKI in the PACU.
- Once decreased urine output or AKI develop, urinary obstruction should be ruled out, and intravascular volume and blood pressure should be restored.
- Intra-abdominal hypertension can compromise renal perfusion despite euvolemia and normotension, increasing the risk of postoperative AKI.

INTRODUCTION

Decreased urine output and acute kidney injury (AKI) are among the most important complications that may develop in the postanesthesia care unit (PACU). Patients with postoperative AKI include those who develop incident kidney disease as well as those with progression of chronic kidney disease. Irrespective of the chronicity of renal impairment, development of AKI is associated with poor patient outcomes.

Funding sources: Dr Chenitz: NIH-NIDDK Training Grant (T32) to the Department of Internal Medicine, University of Pennsylvania (PI: Lawrence Holzman). Dr Lane-Fall: NIH-NHLBI Training Grant (T32) to the Department of Anesthesiology and Critical Care, University of Pennsylvania (PI: David Asch).
Conflicts of interest: None.
[a] Renal, Electrolyte and Hypertension Division, Department of Internal Medicine, Hospital of the University of Pennsylvania, 3400 Spruce Street, 1 Founders Building, Philadelphia, PA 19104, USA; [b] Department of Anesthesiology and Critical Care, Hospital of the University of Pennsylvania, 3400 Spruce Street, 680 Dulles Building, Philadelphia, PA 19104, USA
[1] Both authors contributed equally.
* Corresponding author.
E-mail address: Meghan.Lane-Fall@uphs.upenn.edu

Anesthesiology Clin 30 (2012) 513–526
http://dx.doi.org/10.1016/j.anclin.2012.07.004
1932-2275/12/$ – see front matter © 2012 Elsevier Inc. All rights reserved.

Development of AKI is associated with longer hospital stays[1] and increased in-hospital and overall mortality (25%–90%)[2–4] when compared with patients who do not develop AKI. Due to the deleterious effects of declining renal function, there is an urgent need to prevent the development of AKI. Should AKI develop in the postoperative period, it is equally important to recognize it early and begin appropriate management. This article begins by defining decreased urine output, oliguria, and AKI. It then discusses the epidemiology and risk factors for development of AKI, followed by recommendations for the AKI prevention. Next, the article summarizes the pathophysiology and differential diagnosis of the most common etiologies of decreased urine output and AKI in the PACU. It concludes by presenting diagnostic strategies and management considerations.

DEFINITIONS: DECREASED URINE OUTPUT, OLIGURIA, AND AKI
Decreased Urine Output and Oliguria

Historically, oliguria has been defined as urine excretion less than 400 mL/d.[5] Acute Kidney Injury Network (AKIN) and Risk-Injury-Failure-Loss-End-stage renal disease (RIFLE) classifications of acute kidney injury (**Fig. 1**) define oliguria in progressive stages: <0.5 mL/kg/h × 6 hours, <0.5 mL/kg/h × 12 hours, and <0.3 mL/kg/h × 24 hours.[6,7] Technically then, at least 6 hours of decreased urine output are required for designation of oliguria according to AKIN and RIFLE criteria. Studies evaluating the sensitivity and specificity of urine output as a diagnostic and prognostic measure have yielded mixed results.[8,9] Nonetheless, it remains general consensus that <0.5 mL/kg/h defines decreased urine output. In the proper clinical setting therefore, urine output less than 0.5 mL/kg/h of any duration should prompt consideration and evaluation for causes of oliguria or AKI.

Acute Kidney Injury

Before 2004, there was no consensus definition of AKI. There were greater than 35 definitions in the literature, making evidence-based judgments about prevention and therapy difficult.[10] Thus, in 2004 the Acute Dialysis Quality Initiative examined existing data, and where evidence was lacking, sought expert opinion to form a consensus definition of what was then termed acute renal failure (ARF)–the RIFLE classification.[6]

RIFLE (**Fig. 1**) is an acronym that represents 3 measures of renal dysfunction: (1) *risk* of renal dysfunction, (2) *injury* to the kidney, and (3) *failure* of kidney function and 2 outcome measures (1) *loss* of kidney function and (2) *end-stage* renal disease (ESRD). Loss of kidney function is defined as ARF requiring renal replacement therapy (RRT) for over 4 weeks, and ESRD is defined as requiring RRT for over 3 months. The classification scheme includes separate criteria for changes in serum creatinine and urine output, allowing designation of the severity of AKI on the basis of either measure. Whichever criterion leads to the more severe classification is used.[6] In 2006, the RIFLE criteria were validated in a retrospective study of more than 20,000 inpatients. Approximately 20% of the study patients were found to have some degree of renal impairment, and there was an almost linear increase in hospital mortality from normal renal function to failure.[10]

Despite the apparent success of the RIFLE criteria, new data suggested that smaller changes in serum creatinine than previously cited in the RIFLE criteria may be associated with adverse outcomes.[7,11] Thus, experts in the field convened in 2007 to form the Acute Kidney Injury Network (AKIN). ARF was changed to AKI to represent the entire spectrum of renal impairment. The RIFLE criteria were modified to the further refine the definition of AKI. New and broader criteria to diagnose AKI were adopted in

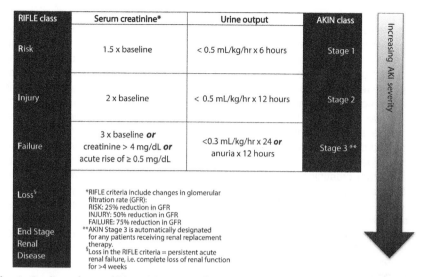

RIFLE class	Serum creatinine*	Urine output	AKIN class
Risk	1.5 x baseline	< 0.5 mL/kg/hr x 6 hours	Stage 1
Injury	2 x baseline	< 0.5 mL/kg/hr x 12 hours	Stage 2
Failure	3 x baseline *or* creatinine > 4 mg/dL *or* acute rise of ≥ 0.5 mg/dL	<0.3 mL/kg/hr x 24 *or* anuria x 12 hours	Stage 3 **
Loss§			
End Stage Renal Disease			

*RIFLE criteria include changes in glomerular filtration rate (GFR):
RISK: 25% reduction in GFR
INJURY: 50% reduction in GFR
FAILURE: 75% reduction in GFR
**AKIN Stage 3 is automatically designated for any patients receiving renal replacement therapy.
§Loss in the RIFLE criteria = persistent acute renal failure, i.e. complete loss of renal function for >4 weeks

Increasing AKI severity

Fig. 1. Grading of acute kidney injury according to RIFLE and AKIN classifications. (*Data from* Bellomo R, Ronco C, Kellum JA, et al. Acute renal failure—definition, outcome measures, animal models, fluid therapy and information technology needs: the Second International Consensus Conference of the Acute Dialysis Quality Initiative (ADQI) Group. Crit Care 2004;8(4):R204–12; and Mehta RL, Kellum JA, Shah SV, et al. Acute kidney injury network: report of an initiative to improve outcomes in acute kidney injury. Crit Care 2007;11:R31.)

efforts to increase clinical awareness and intervention if indicated.[7] Additionally, glomerular filtration rate (GFR) was eliminated as a criterion for renal impairment, because GFR, as calculated by the modification of diet in renal disease (MDRD) equation, has only been validated when renal function is in steady state, not when renal function is in flux as it is in AKI.[8] These changes resulted in a new classification scheme known as the AKIN classification (see **Fig. 1**).

AKIN stages 1, 2, and 3 replace RIFLE's Risk, Injury, and Failure, and patients who require RRT are automatically classified as stage 3. Also, AKIN delineates additional criteria to classify decreased urine output. Urinary tract obstruction must be excluded, and adequate resuscitation must be attempted before applying the diagnostic criteria for decreased urine output. Thus, with this new modification, transient changes in urine output can be excluded.

In studies comparing AKIN with RIFLE, the 2 classifications generally provided similar diagnostic and prognostic value. Despite the modification to RIFLE, AKIN has not been found to improve sensitivity and predictive ability over RIFLE.[8,12,13] Furthermore, in the AKIN scheme, the diagnosis of AKI must be made within a 48-hour timeframe. Thus, if the serum creatinine rises gradually, such as 0.1 mg/dL per day, a slowly progressive AKI would be misclassified.[8,14] Given the variability in designation of AKI in the RIFLE and AKIN classifications, efforts are ongoing to reconcile the 2 schemes and create a single classification universally applicable to the diagnosis of AKI.[8]

EPIDEMIOLOGY AND RISK FACTORS FOR DEVELOPMENT OF POSTOPERATIVE AKI

The risk of developing AKI ranges from 2% to 5% in hospitalized patients[1,15,16] and 1% to 25% in acutely ill patients, depending on the population being studied and the classification used to define AKI.[6] Postsurgical patients may carry even higher risk of decline in renal function than a general inpatient population. Investigators have found a 5% to 10% risk of developing AKI in mixed surgical populations.[17–19] Various factors have been implicated in the risk of postoperative AKI (**Table 1**). In a single-center study, Abelha and colleagues[17] evaluated patients without chronic kidney disease who underwent non-cardiac surgery. They found significant univariate associations between AKI and the following risk factors: age, emergency and high-risk surgery (intraperitoneal, intrathoracic, suprainguinal vascular procedures), ischemic heart disease, congestive heart failure, higher American Society of Anesthesiologists (ASA) physical status, and higher Revised Cardiac Risk Index (RCRI) score. In a different study, perioperative AKI risk factors were examined in the context of cardiothoracic surgery. In a multivariable logistic regression model, age, smoking status, baseline serum creatinine, and diabetes mellitus were found to be preoperative risk factors. Intraoperative risk factors included use of inotropes, erythrocyte transfusion, aortic cross-clamp time, urine output while on cardiopulmonary bypass (CPB), furosemide administration during CPB, and the need for a new CPB pump run. Postoperative AKI risk factors were erythrocyte transfusion and use of vasoconstrictors, inotropes, diuretics, and antiarrhythmic drugs.[19]

CAUSES OF POSTOPERATIVE DECREASED URINE OUTPUT AND ACI

There are myriad causes of decreased urine output and AKI in the postoperative setting. These causes may be divided into those germane to all or most postoperative settings and those unique to specific surgical settings. These two categories will be considered in turn.

Causes of Decreased Urine Output and AKI in a General Postoperative Population

Three broad categories of decreased urine output/AKI etiologies describe the location of the defect in relation to the urogenital system (**Table 2**).

Table 1 Risk factors for development of postoperative AKI	
Preoperative factors	• Preoperative renal dysfunction • Increasing age • Heart disease (ischemic or congestive) • Smoking • Diabetes mellitus • ASA PS 4 or 5
Intraoperative factors	• Emergency surgery, or intraperitoneal, intrathoracic, suprainguinal vascular surgeries • Erythrocyte transfusion • Inotrope use • Aortic cross-clamp time • CPB: furosemide use, urine output, need for a new pump run
Postoperative factors	• Erythrocyte transfusion • Vasoconstrictor use • Diuretic use • Antiarrhythmic drug use

Abbreviations: ASA PS, American Society of Anesthesiologists Physical Status classification; CPB, cardiopulmonary bypass.

Data from Abelha FJ, Botelho M, Fernandes V, et al. Determinants of postoperative acute kidney injury. Crit Care 2009;13(3):R79; and Parolari A, Pesce LL, Pacini D, et al. Risk factors for perioperative acute kidney injury after adult cardiac surgery: role of perioperative management. Ann Thorac Surg 2012;93(2):584–91.

Table 2			
Common causes of postoperative decreased urine output and AKI			
	Site of Defect		
	Prerenal	**Renal**	**Postrenal**

Differential Diagnoses	• Hypotension
	  ○ Absolute
	  ○ Relative
	• Hypovolemia
	  ○ Absolute
	  ○ Relative
	  (eg, IAH)
		• Acute tubular necrosis
		  ○ Ischemia-reperfusion
		  ○ Radiocontrast
		• Acute interstitial nephritis
			• Urinary catheter obstruction
			  ○ Catheter kinking
			  ○ Debris
			• Prostatic hypertrophy
			• Bladder spasm
			• Urinary retention

Abbreviation: IAH, Intra-abdominal hypertension.

Prerenal

Prerenal causes of decreased urine output and AKI include those etiologies that decrease perfusion to the afferent arteriole of the glomerulus. In the postoperative patient, hypotension and hypovolemia are the 2 most important causes of decreased renal perfusion. Either of these phenomena can be absolute or relative.

With regard to hypotension, a mean arterial pressure (MAP) of 60 to 65 mm Hg is usually sufficient to maintain renal perfusion in a patient without pre-existing cardiovascular disease.[20] Lower perfusion pressures may manifest as decreased urine output. Transient hypotension is common in the PACU. In the postoperative patient, euvolemic hypotension may be related to neuraxial analgesia[21] or sedation. Cardiac ischemia or pump failure should be considered as a cause of hypotension, especially in patients with cardiovascular disease. Hypotension accompanied by tachycardia should prompt evaluation for hypovolemia, adrenal insufficiency, and anaphylaxis. Hypotension with bradycardia may indicate beta-blockade, heart block, high neuraxial blockade, or prolonged hypoxemia.

Relative hypotension may occur when patients with pre-existing hypertension exhibit blood pressure values significantly lower than their usual blood pressure. In this setting, maintaining MAP within 20% of baseline should be sufficient to maintain renal perfusion; this is within the range of blood pressure dipping that occurs in most people during sleep.[22]

Hypovolemia may also decrease renal perfusion. Marked hypovolemia is often associated with hypotension, but it is possible to lose in excess of 15% of blood volume before hypotension manifests.[23] Causes of absolute hypovolemia include insufficient replacement of surgical blood loss and dehydration. Dehydration, in turn, may be related to osmotic diuresis (eg, hyperglycemia or mannitol administration), loss of ascites, and preoperative losses such as those caused by vomiting or bowel preparation. Conversely, hypovolemia relative to the kidney may occur in euvolemic or hypervolemic states when renal perfusion is diminished. An important cause of relative hypovolemia in the perioperative setting is intra-abdominal hypertension (IAH). IAH occurs when intra-abdominal pressure increases from a normal value of 5 to 7 mm Hg to values in excess of 12 mm Hg. IAH results from intra-abdominal fluid accumulation and can occur in the setting of edema or intra-abdominal hemorrhage. The elevated abdominal pressure compromises renal preload and afterload, predisposing to renal dysfunction. If intra-abdominal pressure exceeds 20 to 25 mm Hg, frank abdominal compartment syndrome may result, with cardiopulmonary compromise and multiorgan dysfunction.[24]

Renal

Acute tubular necrosis (ATN) is the most important intrarenal cause of AKI in the perioperative setting. ATN, historically characterized by histopathological findings, is now largely a clinical diagnosis.[25] Evidence of renal dysfunction in the appropriate setting is usually sufficient to establish a presumptive diagnosis of ATN. Renal ischemia can cause endothelial and epithelial cell dysfunction that becomes apparent once blood flow is restored. Both apoptotic and immune mechanisms are implicated in the renal dysfunction that follows ischemia and reperfusion.[26] In the perioperative setting, ischemia and reperfusion may occur with peri-procedural systemic hypotension, in the setting of cardiopulmonary bypass,[27] or after aortic cross-clamping for vascular repair[28] or control of hemorrhage. Exposure to nephrotoxins, such as iodinated radiocontrast administered for endovascular procedures, is also associated with ATN.[20]

Acute interstitial nephritis (AIN) is less commonly associated with decreased urine output and AKI in the immediate postoperative period. Nonsteroidal anti-inflammatory drugs (NSAIDs), numerous antibiotics, and diuretics are among the drugs reported to cause drug-induced AIN.[29]

Postrenal

Postrenal causes of decreased urine output and AKI are those causing physical obstruction of the urinary system distal to the renal pelvis. Obstruction may be internal (eg, blood clots, urinary catheter debris) or external to the urethra or urinary catheter (eg, prostatic hypertrophy, urinary catheter kinking). Functional obstruction may occur with conditions impairing bladder emptying, such as neurogenic bladder,[30] bladder spasm or narcotic-related urinary retention.

Procedure-Specific Causes of Postoperative Decreased Urine Output and AKI

In addition to the causes listed previously, it is important to consider how the technical aspects of specific surgical procedures may predispose an at-risk patient to the development of decreased urine output or AKI (**Table 3**).

Urologic surgery

Patients who undergo intra-abdominal urologic surgery such as cystectomy and diversion are at risk for urologic complications related to manipulation of the ureters or anastomosis of the ureters to a urinary reservoir or conduit. These complications are rare in the immediate postoperative period; a retrospective secondary data analysis of 6577 patients in the United States undergoing radical cystectomy showed

Table 3
Selected procedure-specific causes of decreased urine output and AKI

Surgical Specialty	Example of Procedure	Connection to AKI
Urology	Cystectomy and diversion	Ureteral damage, compromised ureteral anastomoses
General surgery and gynecology	Colectomy, hysterectomy	Ureteral damage
Cardiac surgery	Any procedure with CPB	Acute tubular necrosis from ischemia–reperfusion, nonpulsatile flow, complement activation
Vascular surgery	Endovascular aortic aneurysm repair	Renal ischemia from partial or complete stenting over the renal arteries, contrast-induced nephropathy

a urinary complication rate of 2.92%.[31] A more recent large single-center prospective observational study showed a genitourinary (GU) complication rate less than 7% in the 30 days following surgery that increased over time. The types of GU complications encountered included acute renal failure or worsening of pre-existing renal insufficiency, urinary infections, ureteral stenosis, and hydronephrosis.[32] When evaluating the urine output of a patient after cystectomy, it is important to note urine excretion may occur via an abdominal urostomy or continent cutaneous diversion.[33] A urethral catheter in this setting may be left as a pelvic drain but will not drain urine. Ultimately, the patient's GU anatomy should be clarified with the surgical team.

General and gynecologic surgery

Any intra-abdominal procedure in the lower abdomen or pelvis presents a risk for ureteral injury. Placement of ureteral stents for intraoperative ureteral identification is common, but does not eliminate the risk of ureteral injury.[34] In a recent single-center study of more than 5000 colorectal surgery patients, ureteral injury was noted in 14 patients. Half of the patients had ureteral stents placed. In 2 of the 14 patients, the presenting symptoms were anuria (1 patient) and acute renal failure (1 patient) on postoperative day 1.[35]

Cardiac surgery

Despite the increasing use of fast-track anesthesia and extubation in the operating room for patients receiving coronary artery bypass grafting, most cardiac surgery patients are admitted postoperatively to an intensive care unit for close monitoring.[36] If postoperative cardiac surgery patients are encountered in the PACU, they may be at risk for AKI as a result of ischemia–reperfusion injury or complement activation by the cardiopulmonary bypass circuit.[27]

Vascular surgery

Open abdominal aortic aneurysm repair may be associated with ureteral injury, as discussed previously for general and gynecologic surgery. Ischemia–reperfusion and dislodgement of atheromatous plaques by aortic cross-clamping are also important factors in AKI following aortic aneurysm repair.[28] In contrast, endovascular stenting of aortic aneurysms is associated with decreased risk of AKI,[28] but intraoperative contrast load and renal artery occlusion by the aortic stent are unique mechanisms leading to kidney injury.[37]

PREVENTION OF AKI

As mentioned earlier, it is preferable to avoid development of AKI in the postoperative period. There are several types of interventions that have been studied for their potential to help avoid development of postoperative AKI: monitoring, fluid therapy, vasopressor therapy, avoidance of intra-abdominal hypertension, avoidance of contrast-induced nephropathy, and pharmacologic interventions. Each of these types of interventions will be considered in turn.

Monitoring

As discussed previously, postoperative AKI may be related to perioperative renal hypoperfusion and ischemic injury as a consequence of hemodynamic instability resulting from hypovolemia, hypotension, or decreased cardiac output. As such, it is reasonable to consider whether aggressive hemodynamic monitoring is beneficial. However, a preferred method of hemodynamic monitoring to prevent development of AKI has yet to be determined.[38] A randomized control trial evaluated the use pulmonary artery catheters in high-risk surgical patients, and found no benefit in prevention of AKI.[39] Nevertheless, use of these catheters remains commonplace when cardiac output is uncertain.[38] Less invasive cardiac monitoring techniques such as pulse pressure variation and use of esophageal Doppler probes are increasingly used for perioperative hemodynamic management,[38,40] but it is not clear whether use of these methods protects against development of postoperative AKI.

Fluid Therapy

The administration of fluid to restore intravascular volume is a mainstay of therapy in preventing AKI, although the optimal amount of fluid therapy is unclear. Lopes and colleagues[41] demonstrated that intraoperative fluid boluses titrated in accordance with the variation in arterial pulse pressure improve postoperative outcomes. However, Bouchard and colleagues[42] demonstrated that fluid accumulation in critically ill patients with acute illness is associated with increased mortality, and is not associated with recovery of renal function. Furthermore, liberal fluid administration in patients undergoing bowel surgery has been associated with increased cardiopulmonary and tissue-healing complications, arguing for restricted fluid therapy in this context.[43]

There is also controversy surrounding fluid choice in volume resuscitation. Colloids have been shown to more effectively increase cardiac filling,[44] but an overall mortality benefit of colloids in comparison to crystalloids has not been demonstrated.[28] Hydroxyethyl starch, a synthetic colloid, has been shown in multiple studies, including several randomized control trials, to be nephrotoxic.[45] Use of blood as a resuscitation fluid is also not without risk. As mentioned previously, erythrocyte infusion has been shown to be independently associated with the development of AKI in cardiothoracic surgery.[19]

Fluid therapy in the setting of cardiopulmonary bypass has also been studied. Haase and colleagues[46] proposed that 1 of the potential etiologies of CPB-associated AKI is urinary acidity leading to toxicity from reactive oxygen species and complement activation. To answer this question, this group conducted a pilot study determining whether urinary alkalization is renoprotective in patients undergoing CPB. The study concluded that load and continuous administration of sodium bicarbonate in patients undergoing CPB reduces the risk of AKI. This finding has yet to be validated in larger trials.

Vasopressor therapy

In efforts to reduce the risk of AKI, it is necessary to maintain adequate renal perfusion pressures. Once intravascular volume has been restored with fluid administration, if the patient continues to have arterial hypotension, administration of vasoconstricting medication is indicated. The mainstay of clinical practice is to keep the mean arterial pressure above 60 to 65 mm Hg, but patients with renovascular disease or long-standing hypertension may require higher arterial pressures to maintain renal perfusion.[20]

Avoidance or Treatment of Intra-Abdominal Hypertension

Another cause of decreased renal perfusion is intra-abdominal hypertension, discussed previously as 1 of the causes of decreased urine output and AKI. Several conditions can cause elevated abdominal pressures, such as blood or ascites accumulation in the abdomen, distended bowel, or operative abdominal closure with edematous bowel, in the setting of a noncompliant abdominal wall.[47] Abdominal pressure can be measured through bladder catheter transduction. Once abdominal hypertension is identified, procedural intervention to decrease abdominal pressures, such as therapeutic paracentesis or exploratory laparotomy, may prevent AKI.[20]

Avoidance of Contrast-Induced Nephropathy

Intravenous fluids given before, during, and after the administration of iodinated contrast have been shown to reduce the risk of contrast-induced nephropathy (CIN).[48] Thus, fluid administration is recommended during procedures involving the use of intravenous iodinated contrast agents, such as endovascular procedures. However, the optimal type of fluid—sodium bicarbonate, normal saline, or other isotonic crystalloid solutions—remains controversial. In patients undergoing coronary angiography, intravenous sodium bicarbonate was shown to reduce the risk of CIN as compared with normal saline, but there was no improvement in hospital length of stay or mortality.[49] As intravenous fluids are beneficial in the prevention of CIN, diuretics and volume depletion pose potential risk and should be avoided.[20] Studies evaluating N-acetylcysteine in the prevention of CIN yielded mixed results.[49]

Pharmacologic Interventions

Both dopamine and atrial natriuretic peptide (ANP) initially showed promise in the prevention of AKI due to their vasoactive effects leading to increased renal blood flow. Although evidence suggests ANP may reduce the necessity for RRT, neither dopamine nor ANP was associated with improved mortality. Likewise fenoldopam, a selective dopamine receptor agonist, initially showed potential for renoprotective benefit. In large studies, however, fenoldopam was not shown to be beneficial in prevention of AKI.[50–52]

In summary, prevention of postoperative AKI should include optimization of renal perfusion by managing hemodynamics, intravascular volume, and avoiding increases in intra-abdominal pressure. Administering fluids in the setting of radiocontrast exposure may prevent development of AKI. Although not explored here, it is also prudent to avoid administration of nephrotoxins such as NSAIDs, aminoglycosides, and tacrolimus, when possible, in patients who have risk factors for development of postoperative AKI.

PRESENTATION OF DECREASED URINE OUTPUT AND AKI IN THE PACU

As discussed earlier, the term oliguria refers to decreased urine output that has persisted for at least 6 to 24 hours.[6] The term "decreased urine output" is used here to describe the decreases in urine output that are likely to be seen in the PACU patient, whose average length of stay is insufficient to allow diagnosis of oliguria. Urine output of less than 30 mL/h (roughly 0.5 mL/kg/h for a 70 kg patient) should be considered cause for concern.

Recognition of decreased urine output is much more straightforward than recognition of AKI in the PACU. For patients receiving postoperative laboratory studies, AKI may manifest as increased blood urea nitrogen (BUN) and creatinine, with or without decrease in urine output. According to RIFLE criteria, a 50% increase in creatinine places the patient at risk of AKI.[6] If preoperative creatinine values are not available, it is important to remember that serum creatinine must be interpreted with the patient's age, sex, and body weight in mind. Normal creatinine (corresponding to GFR >100 mL/min) for a 20-year-old 70 kg man is roughly 1.0 mg/dL based on the MDRD equation; a normal value for a 90-year-old 50 kg woman is 0.6 mg/dL.[53]

More rarely, patients with severe AKI in the PACU may exhibit signs of florid renal failure that usually constitute indications for urgent renal replacement therapy: volume overload leading to congestive heart failure and pulmonary edema, hyperkalemia, and acidemia.[54] Postoperative patients are unlikely to acutely demonstrate other indications for urgent dialysis, including hypermagnesemia and symptomatic uremia.

DIAGNOSIS OF DECREASED URINE OUTPUT AND AKI IN THE PACU

The evaluation of decreased urine output and AKI in the PACU should be guided by the patient's history and presentation. As mentioned earlier, hypotension and hypovolemia are important causes of AKI. It is important to approach diagnosis of decreased urine output and AKI in a stepwise fashion, considering the most common and most easily remedied causes first. An example of a diagnostic algorithm is presented in (**Fig. 2**).

MANAGEMENT OF DECREASED URINE OUTPUT AND AKI IN THE PACU

Determining the etiology of AKI is the initial step in management.[55] Once reversible causes of AKI such as obstruction, hypotension, hypovolemia and intra-abdominal hypertension are excluded or ameliorated, the fundamental strategy for renal protection in the early stages of AKI continues to be maintenance of adequate renal perfusion and minimization of nephrotoxins.[52] Renal perfusion may be maintained with fluid administration or vasoactive medication, but as discussed previously, the amount of fluid or the selection of the type of fluid or vasoactive medication has not been established.

What is the role for pharmacologic treatment of postoperative AKI? The use of diuretics in the management of AKI in general is historically contested. Oliguria has been associated with increased mortality in patients with AKI[56]; it also makes fluid balance difficult to achieve. Animal models support the use of diuretics in AKI. The kidney demands a certain amount of oxygen to reabsorb sodium. Since loop diuretics block sodium reabsorption, experimental evidence has suggested that they also increase oxygen generation in renal tissue thereby reducing the risk of AKI.[57] Also in

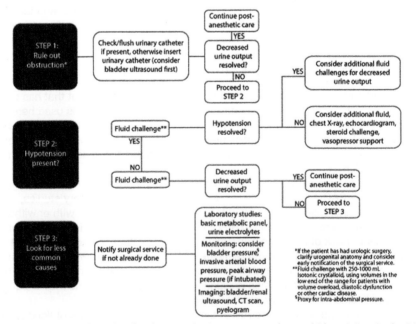

Fig. 2. Diagnostic algorithm for decreased urine output and acute kidney injury in the PACU.

animal models, loop diuretics have been shown to improve renal blood flow by decreasing renal vascular resistance. However, in clinical trials, the use of diuretics in AKI failed to show any significant benefit in clinical outcome. Thus, diuretics may be useful in maintaining fluid balance, but they are not an effective treatment for AKI itself. Moreover, hypovolemia with diuretic use must be avoided so as not to compound renal injury.[57] Other pharmacologic interventions such as dopamine or ANP have not been shown to improve outcomes in AKI.[52]

Once the diagnosis of renal failure has been made, and reversible causes treated, the management plan must then be focused on minimizing the complications associated with renal failure. Weight and fluid intake should be strictly recorded; serum chemistries should be drawn assess for metabolic disarray. If profound hyperkalemia, metabolic acidosis, or volume overload is detected, renal replacement therapy may be indicated (**Fig. 2**).[58]

SUMMARY

Decreased urine output (urine output less than 0.5 mL/kg/h) is commonly encountered in the PACU. AKI in the PACU is rarer, but development of AKI is a very poor prognostic sign. Prevention of AKI is optimal, but once it has developed, rapid recognition and supportive treatment are important to optimize patient outcomes. The mainstay of supportive therapy for decreased urine output and AKI is restoration of intravascular volume and renal blood flow. Pharmacologic treatment and renal replacement therapy are usually not indicated for treatment of decreased urine output and AKI in the immediate postoperative setting.

REFERENCES

1. Chertow GM, Burdick E, Honour M, et al. Acute kidney injury, mortality, length of stay, and costs in hospitalized patients. J Am Soc Nephrol 2005;16(11):3365–70.
2. Carmichael P, Carmichael AR. Acute renal failure in the surgical setting. ANZ J Surg 2003;73(3):144–53.
3. Ishani A, Nelson D, Clothier B, et al. The magnitude of acute serum creatinine increase after cardiac surgery and the risk of chronic kidney disease, progression of kidney disease, and death. Arch Intern Med 2011;171(3):226–33.
4. Levy EM, Viscoli CM, Horwitz RI. The effect of acute renal failure on mortality: a cohort analysis. J Am Med Assoc 1996;275(19):1489–94.
5. Klahr S, Miller SB. Acute oliguria. N Engl J Med 1998;338(10):671–5.
6. Bellomo R, Ronco C, Kellum JA, et al. Acute renal failure—definition, outcome measures, animal models, fluid therapy and information technology needs: the second international consensus conference of the Acute Dialysis Quality Initiative (ADQI) group. Crit Care 2004;8(4):R204–12.
7. Mehta RL, Kellum JA, Shah SV, et al. Acute kidney injury network: report of an initiative to improve outcomes in acute kidney injury. Crit Care 2007;11:R31.
8. Cruz DN, Ricci Z, Ronco C. Clinical review: RIFLE and AKIN–time for reappraisal. Crit Care 2009;13(3):211.
9. Macedo E, Malhotra R, Bouchard J, et al. Oliguria is an early predictor of higher mortality in critically ill patients. Kidney 2011;80(7):760–7.
10. Uchino S, Bellomo R, Goldsmith D, et al. An assessment of the RIFLE criteria for acute renal failure in hospitalized patients. Crit Care Med 2006;34(7):1913–7.
11. Lassnigg A, Schmidlin D, Mouhieddine M, et al. Minimal changes of serum creatinine predict prognosis in patients after cardiothoracic surgery: a prospective cohort study. J Am Soc Nephrol 2004;15(6):1597–605.

12. Bagshaw SM, George C, Bellomo R, et al. A comparison of the RIFLE and AKIN criteria for acute kidney injury in critically ill patients. Nephrol Dial Transplant 2008;23(5):1569–74.

13. Haase M, Bellomo R, Matalanis G, et al. A comparison of the RIFLE and Acute Kidney Injury Network classifications for cardiac surgery-associated acute kidney injury: a prospective cohort study. J Thorac Cardiovasc Surg 2009;138(6): 1370–6.

14. Ostermann M. Acute kidney injury on admission to the intensive care unit: where to go from here? Crit Care 2008;12(6):189.

15. Kheterpal S, Tremper KK, Englesbe MJ, et al. Predictors of postoperative acute renal failure after noncardiac surgery in patients with previously normal renal function. Anesthesiology 2007;107(6):892–902.

16. Shusterman N, Strom BL, Murray TG, et al. Risk factors and outcome of hospital-acquired acute renal failure. Clinical epidemiologic study. Am J Med 1987;83(1):65–71.

17. Abelha FJ, Botelho M, Fernandes V, et al. Determinants of postoperative acute kidney injury. Crit Care 2009;13(3):R79.

18. Shaw A, Swaminathan M, Stafford-Smith M. Cardiac surgery-associated acute kidney injury: putting together the pieces of the puzzle. Nephron Physiol 2008; 109(4):p55–60.

19. Parolari A, Pesce LL, Pacini D, et al. Risk factors for perioperative acute kidney injury after adult cardiac surgery: role of perioperative management. Ann Thorac Surg 2012;93(2):584–91.

20. Venkataraman R, Kellum JA. Prevention of acute renal failure. Chest 2007;131(1): 300–8.

21. Bauer M, George JE III, Seif J, et al. Recent advances in epidural analgesia. Anesthesiol Res Pract 2012;2012:309219.

22. Loredo JS, Nelesen R, Ancoli-Israel S, et al. Sleep quality and blood pressure dipping in normal adults. Sleep 2004;27(6):1097–103.

23. Gutierrez G, Reines HD, Wulf-Gutierrez ME. Clinical review: hemorrhagic shock. Crit Care 2004;8(5):373–81.

24. Ameloot K, Gillebert C, Desie N, et al. Hypoperfusion, shock states, and abdominal compartment syndrome (ACS). Surg Clin North Am 2012;92(2):207–20.

25. Kellum JA. Acute kidney injury. Crit Care Med 2008;36(Suppl 4):S141–5.

26. Kinsey GR, Okusa MD. Pathogenesis of acute kidney injury: foundation for clinical practice. Am J Kidney Dis 2011;58(2):291–301.

27. Diaz GC, Moitra V, Sladen RN. Hepatic and renal protection during cardiac surgery. Anesthesiol Clin 2008;26(3):565–90.

28. Wald R, Waikar SS, Liangos O, et al. Acute renal failure after endovascular vs open repair of abdominal aortic aneurysm. J Vasc Surg 2006;43(3):460–6.

29. Kodner CM, Kudrimoti A. Diagnosis and management of acute interstitial nephritis. Am Fam Physician 2003;67(12):2527–39.

30. Tseng TY, Stoller ML. Obstructive uropathy. Clin Geriatr Med 2009;25(3):437–43.

31. Konety BR, Allareddy V, Herr H. Complications after radical cystectomy: analysis of population-based data. Urology 2006;68(1):58–64.

32. Shabsigh A, Korets R, Vora KC, et al. Defining early morbidity of radical cystectomy for patients with bladder cancer using a standardized reporting methodology. Eur Urol 2009;55(1):164–76.

33. Konety BR, Barbour S, Carroll PR. Urinary diversion and bladder substitution. In: Tanagho EA, McAninch JW, editors. Smith's general urology. 17th edition. New York: McGraw-Hill; 2008. Available at: http://www.accessmedicine.com/content.aspx?aID=3128758. Accessed June 26, 2012.

34. Brandes S, Coburn M, Armenakas N, et al. Diagnosis and management of ureteric injury: an evidence-based analysis. BJU Int 2004;94(3):277–89.
35. Palaniappa NC, Telem DA, Ranasinghe NE, et al. Incidence of iatrogenic ureteral injury after laparoscopic colectomy. Arch Surg 2012;147(3):267–71.
36. Van Mastrigt GA, Heijmans J, Severens JL, et al. Short-stay intensive care after coronary artery bypass surgery: randomized clinical trial on safety and cost-effectiveness. Crit Care Med 2006;34(1):65–75.
37. Maleux G, Koolen M, Heye S. Complications after endovascular aneurysm repair. Semin Intervent Radiol 2009;26(1):3–9.
38. Schetz M, Bove T, Morelli A, et al. Prevention of cardiac surgery-associated acute kidney injury. Int J Artif Organs 2008;31(2):179–89.
39. Sandham JD, Hull RD, Brant RF, et al. A randomized, controlled trial of the use of pulmonary-artery catheters in high-risk surgical patients. N Engl J Med 2003; 348(1):5–14.
40. Marquez J, McCurry K, Severyn DA, et al. Ability of pulse power, esophageal Doppler, and arterial pulse pressure to estimate rapid changes in stroke volume in humans. Crit Care Med 2008;36(11):3001–7.
41. Lopes MR, Oliveira MA, Pereira VO, et al. Goal-directed fluid management based on pulse pressure variation monitoring during high-risk surgery: a pilot randomized controlled trial. Crit Care 2007;11(5):R100.
42. Bouchard J, Soroko SB, Chertow GM, et al. Fluid accumulation, survival and recovery of kidney function in critically ill patients with acute kidney injury. Kidney 2009;76(4):422–7.
43. Brandstrup B, Tonnesen H, Beier-Holgersen R, et al. Effects of intravenous fluid restriction on postoperative complications: comparison of two perioperative fluid regimens: a randomized assessor-blinded multicenter trial. Ann Surg 2003; 238(5):641–8.
44. Trof RJ, Sukul SP, Twisk JW, et al. Greater cardiac response of colloid than saline fluid loading in septic and non-septic critically ill patients with clinical hypovolaemia. Intensive Care Med 2010;36(4):697–701.
45. Groeneveld AB, Navickis RJ, Wilkes MM. Update on the comparative safety of colloids: a systematic review of clinical studies. Ann Surg 2011;253(3):470–83.
46. Haase M, Haase-Fielitz A, Bellomo R, et al. Sodium bicarbonate to prevent increases in serum creatinine after cardiac surgery: a pilot double-blind, randomized controlled trial. Crit Care Med 2009;37(1):39–47.
47. Malbrain ML, Chiumello D, Pelosi P, et al. Incidence and prognosis of intraabdominal hypertension in a mixed population of critically ill patients: a multiple-center epidemiological study. Crit Care Med 2005;33(2):315–22.
48. Rudnick MR, Kesselheim A, Goldfarb S. Contrast-induced nephropathy: how it develops, how to prevent it. Cleve Clin J Med 2006;73(1):75–80, 83–7.
49. Navaneethan SD, Singh S, Appasamy S, et al. Sodium bicarbonate therapy for prevention of contrast-induced nephropathy: a systematic review and meta-analysis. Am J Kidney Dis 2009;53(4):617–27.
50. Nigwekar SU, Navaneethan SD, Parikh CR, et al. Atrial natriuretic peptide for management of acute kidney injury: a systematic review and meta-analysis. Clin J Am Soc Nephrol 2009;4(2):261–72.
51. Friedrich JO, Adhikari N, Herridge MS, et al. Meta-analysis: low-dose dopamine increases urine output but does not prevent renal dysfunction or death. Ann Intern Med 2005;142(7):510–24.
52. Tolwani A, Paganini E, Joannidis M, et al. Treatment of patients with cardiac surgery associated-acute kidney injury. Int J Artif Organs 2008;31(2):190–6.

53. Roth D, Rogers N, Greene T, et al. A more accurate method to estimate glomerular filtration rate from serum creatinine: a new prediction equation. Ann Intern Med 1999;130(6):461–70.
54. Gibney N, Hoste E, Burdmann EA, et al. Timing of initiation and discontinuation of renal replacement therapy in AKI: unanswered key questions. Clin J Am Soc Nephrol 2008;3(3):876–80.
55. Sykes E, Cosgrove JF. Acute renal failure and the critically ill surgical patient. Ann R Coll Surg Engl 2007;89(1):22–9.
56. Bagshaw SM, Bellomo R, Kellum JA. Oliguria, volume overload, and loop diuretics. Crit Care Med 2008;36(Suppl 4):S172–8.
57. Nigwekar SU, Waikar SS. Diuretics in acute kidney injury. Semin Nephrol 2011;31(6):523–34.
58. Palevsky PM. Indications and timing of renal replacement therapy in acute kidney injury. Crit Care Med 2008;36(Suppl 4):S224–8.

Hemodynamic and Related Challenges

Monitoring and Regulation in the Postoperative Period

Andrew Plante, MD, Eliot Ro, MD, James R. Rowbottom, MD*

KEYWORDS

- Postoperative complications • Postoperative oliguria • Hemodynamic complications
- Postoperative arrhythmia • Postoperative hypotension • Postoperative hypothermia
- Postoperative monitoring modalities • PACU

KEY POINTS

- Airway obstruction in the postoperative period is a common complication necessitating early intervention to maintain oxygenation and ventilation in the recovering patient.
- The potential causes of postoperative hypotension are diverse, but the risk of inadequate tissue perfusion has a common end point: shock.
- The implications of hypothermia on perioperative hemodynamics include increased SVR, myocardial irritability, and susceptibility to arrhythmias as well as coagulopathy.
- Perioperative arrhythmias may have significant effects on myocardial O_2 supply and demand and the resultant hemodynamic profile.
- Postoperative oliguria is a sensitive indicator of end organ perfusion as it may reflect simple hypovolemia or severe hemodynamic compromise.

INTRODUCTION

The aging population with significant comorbidities has necessitated improved capabilities of caring for patients in the postoperative period. The immediate postoperative period poses unique challenges to caregivers. Approximately 23.7% of patients admitted to the post anesthesia care unit (PACU) experience problems that affect their postoperative course (the most frequent are nausea and vomiting, 9.8%; upper airway obstruction, 6.9%; and hypotension, 2.7%).[1] Although frequently managed effectively, the cause is often difficult to identify and occasionally represents an early manifestation of an evolving disease process. Great progress to ensure patient safety has been made, and increasing accuracy of diagnostic skills, evaluation, and monitoring

Department of Anesthesiology & Perioperative Medicine, University Hospitals, Case Medical Center, 11100 Euclid Avenue, Cleveland, OH 44106, USA
* Corresponding author.
E-mail address: james.rowbottom1@uhhospitals.org

Anesthesiology Clin 30 (2012) 527–554
http://dx.doi.org/10.1016/j.anclin.2012.07.012
1932-2275/12/$ – see front matter © 2012 Elsevier Inc. All rights reserved.

modalities is enabling high-quality care and improved outcomes. This article presents several common challenges seen in the immediate postoperative period, reviews their physiologic basis and effects on postoperative hemodynamics, and discusses evaluation and monitoring options to facilitate optimal outcomes.

Postoperative monitoring of patients is based on the fundamental American Society of Anesthesiologists (ASA) standards.[2] Establishing these as the minimum standard for patient care has helped ensure improved patient safety and decreased morbidity and mortality.[3] Applying these monitors in the immediate postoperative period and extending into the perioperative period further contributes to enhanced safety.

Clinicians continue to see development of improved diagnostic and monitoring devices, with an emphasis on decreasing invasiveness and subsequent risk to patients. Despite a large arsenal of tools, a logical approach and plan for use must be devised to achieve maximal benefit. Cost is always a consideration because expensive new technology is being introduced into practice, seemingly on a daily basis.

This article does not promote a particular product, brand, or monitoring device, but proposes an approach to caring for patients in the critical immediate postoperative period. It begins with the following scenario:

A 75-year-old woman presented with a history of insulin-dependent diabetes mellitus (IDDM), obstructive sleep apnea (OSA), chronic obstructive pulmonary disease (COPD), coronary artery disease (CAD) with myocardial infraction (MI) 5 years ago, ischemic cardiomyopathy (ICM), and mild chronic renal insufficiency (CRI) with a baseline creatinine (CR) of 1.6. Her medications include an albuterol inhaler, aspirin, metoprolol, insulin, lisinopril, furosemide, and multivitamins. She presented to the emergency department with a 72-hour history of nausea, lower abdominal pain, and low-grade fever. Her evaluation included a history and physical examination with vital signs (temperature [T] 38°C, heart rate [HR] 90 beats per minute [bpm], respiratory rate [RR] 24, blood pressure [BP] 136/82 mm Hg, and pulse oximeter [Spo_2] oxygen saturation of 97%), complete blood count (CBC) with differential, basic metabolic panel (BMP), electrocardiogram (ECG) sinus rhythm (SR) with Q waves inferiorly, and a computed tomography (CT) scan of the abdomen and pelvis with oral and intravenous (IV) contrast that was suspicious for appendicitis. She was urgently taken to the operating room for a laparoscopic appendectomy (**Table 1**).

The patient underwent an uncomplicated, 60-minute procedure using general anesthesia (GA; rapid sequence induction [RSI], oral endotracheal tube [OETT], propofol, rocuronium, fentanyl, midazolam, sevoflurane, neostigmine and glycopyrrolate) using ASA standard monitors for the procedure. She was hemodynamically stable (vital signs within 20% of baseline parameters); had minimal blood loss (75 mL); received

Table 1 Patient work-up	
Past Medical History	**Medications**
IDDM	Insulin
COPD	Albuterol
CAD	Aspirin
MI	Metoprolol
ICM	Lisinopril
CRI	Furosemide
OSA	—

1500 mL of crystalloid IV fluids and had 50 mL of urine output. The findings on laparoscopy included a ruptured appendix that necessitated extending one of the incisions for improved access and copious irrigation. At the end of the procedure, after noting 3 twitches on the train-of-four (TOF) monitor, paralysis was reversed with weight-appropriate doses of neostigmine and glycopyrrolate. After meeting extubation criteria, the OETT was removed and the patient was taken to the PACU.

On arrival in the PACU, monitors were applied with admitting vital signs of T, 35.2°C; P, 108 bpm; RR, 26; BP, 170/ 92 mm Hg; and Spo_2, 92% on a simple face mask at 10 L/min oxygen (O_2) flow. She was snoring loudly and was difficult to arouse. Her glucose was 200 g/dL.

The patient encountered several common problems during her PACU stay. This article reviews her course with an emphasis on differential diagnosis, evaluation strategies, and monitoring options (with a comparison of modalities), and proposes a rationale for treatment.

AIRWAY OBSTRUCTION

Establishing the airway is a primary step in the management of operative and critically ill patients. This focus implies an importance beyond providing a conduit, but enables oxygenation and ventilation that support aerobic metabolism and cell survival. The impact of these basic functions on hemodynamics is reviewed.

Oxygenation

Hypoxemia is defined as low O_2 content in the blood, whereas hypoxia is inadequate tissue oxygenation. Oxygen availability to the tissues depends on 3 main factors:

Oxygen content of blood
Oxygen content of blood depends on O_2 bound to hemoglobin (Hb) and dissolved in the blood. Causes of hypoxemia are listed in **Table 2**.

$$\text{Oxygen Content of Blood } (Cao_2) = 1.34 \, (Hb)(O_2 \text{ sat}) + (0.003)(Pao_2)$$

Table 2 Causes of hypoxemia	
Causes of Hypoxemia	**Comment[37,38]**
Low Fio_2	High altitude
Low diffusion of O_2 into blood	Capillary diffusion abnormality CO_2 diffuses 20 times faster than O_2
Hypoventilation	Increased CO_2 displaces O_2 in alveoli (described by alveolar gas equation)
Ventilation-perfusion mismatch (V/Q)	Mismatch in areas of diseased or damaged lung: fat emboli and pulmonary embolus Improves with supplemental O_2
Shunt	Venous blood passes through lung without increasing oxygen content Occurs with pulmonary edema, atelectasis and consolidation. No improvement with supplemental O_2

Abbreviation: Fio_2, inspired O_2 fraction.

Oxygen delivery

Oxygen delivery depends on cardiac output and Cao_2.

$$CO = HR \times stroke\ volume\ (SV)$$

$$Oxygen\ delivery\ (DO_2) = CO \times Cao_2 \times 10\ (conversion\ factor)$$

Oxygen use by tissues

The basal metabolic rate is 3 mL/kg/min, and is increased in hypermetabolic states. Oxygen must be delivered and released for use by the tissues. The oxyhemoglobin dissociation curve explains the loading and unloading of O_2 from Hb (**Fig. 1**).

Ventilation

Carbon dioxide (CO_2) is produced at the same rate that O_2 is consumed and increases with increasing metabolic activity. It is freely diffusible and is eliminated by the lungs except for a residual amount in the alveoli and in blood ($\sim$40 mm Hg). Ventilation is expressed as:

$$Minute\ Ventilation\ (V_E) = RR \times Tidal\ Volume\ (TV)$$

V_E is the respiratory mechanism to control acid-base balance. Hypoventilation increases CO_2, which creates a respiratory acidosis or may exacerbate a metabolic acidosis. Abnormal pH has hemodynamic implications, as noted in **Box 1**. CO_2 also affects oxygenation. The profound effects of these respiratory abnormalities on hemodynamics are summarized in **Table 3**.

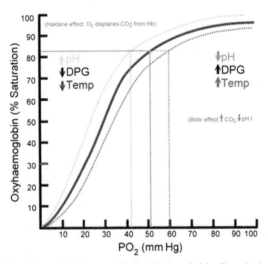

Fig. 1. Oxyhemoglobin dissociation curve. The oxyhemoglobin dissociation curve details the cooperative binding and unloading of oxygen from Hb. The conditions that affect the cooperative binding shift the curve. Right shift indicates decreased affinity of Hb for oxygen, which promotes unloading of oxygen to the tissues; left shift indicates increased affinity of Hb for oxygen, so less oxygen is released to the tissues. DPG, Diphosphoglycerate. (*From* Wikipedia contributors. Oxyhaemoglobin dissociation curve. Available at: http://en.wikipedia.org/wiki/File:Oxyhaemoglobin_dissociation_curve.png.)

Box 1
Hemodynamic effects of acidosis

Hypoxemia

↓ Contractility

Hypotension

Right shift of the oxyhemoglobin dissociation curve

↓ Response to catecholamines

Tissue hypoxia (despite ↑ O_2 unloading in tissues)

↓ Threshold for ventricular fibrillation

Hyperkalemia

Data from Morgan GE Jr, Mikhail MS, Murray MJ. Chapter 30. Acid–base balance. In: Morgan GE Jr, Mikhail MS, Murray MJ, editors. Clinical anesthesiology. 4th edition New York: McGraw-Hill; 2006.

Airway obstruction is a common postoperative finding and is usually caused by collapse of the upper airway. Common causes for obstruction are listed in **Table 4**.

Evaluation should always begin with a focused physical examination for respiratory effort, chest rise, air movement and accessory muscle use. Assessment of mental status can also provide valuable clues to the cause of the respiratory failure. An alert patient with airway obstruction is more likely to have upper airway edema, obstructive sputum, a foreign body, recurrent laryngeal nerve injury, or damage to the vocal cords (especially after head and neck surgery). Stridor is an abnormal inspiratory breath sound that often accompanies upper airway obstruction. Assessment of muscle strength includes hand grasp, head lift, and TOF testing. Beyond the physical examination, monitoring is accomplished by the use of pulse oximetry. Capnography or other methods of monitoring expired CO_2 may also be indicated.

Treatment of obstruction often consists of a simple jaw thrust and placement of an oral or nasal airway to displace the tongue and soft palate. If the patient has known

---

Table 3
Hemodynamic effects of oxygenation and ventilation abnormalities

Hypoxemia	Hypercarbia	Hypocarbia
↑ HR	↓ Myocardial contractility and vasodilation causes ↑ sympathetic nervous system activity with resultant ↑ cardiac output, HR, and BP	Vasoconstriction
↑ cardiac output		
↓ SVR, but stable blood pressure		
Hypoxic pulmonary vasoconstriction: optimize V/Q matching	Vasodilation	
Pulmonary hypertension	Coronary vasodilation	
	Arrhythmias from ↑ catecholamines	

Abbreviation: SVI, systemic vascular resistance.

Data from Patel PM, Patel HH, Roth DM. Chapter 19. General anesthetics and therapeutic gases. In: Brunton LL, Chabner BA, Knollmann BC, editors. Goodman & Gilman's the pharmacologic basis of therapeutics. 12th edition New York: McGraw-Hill; 2011.

Table 4
Airway obstruction (the second most common PACU complication,[1] occurring in 6.9%–8.5% of all PACU admissions[1,39])

Airway Obstruction

In general:
~50% can be managed with a nasal airway[1]
~25% require pharyngeal airway support[1]
~0.2% require reintubation[39].
- 77% within 1 h of extubation or PACU admission
- 54% in patients >60 y of age
- 23% following ear, nose, and throat procedures

Unanticipated early (within 72 h) postoperative intubation occurs in 0.83%–0.9% of patients (independent predictor of 30-d mortality)[40]

Differential Diagnosis	Clinical Signs and Symptoms	Vital Signs	Monitors	Laboratory Tests	Treatment
Residual anesthetic	Sedated or cannot be aroused	T $\leftrightarrow$	Pulse oximeter	ABG: $Pao_2 \downarrow$, $Pco_2 \uparrow$, pH	Chin lift/jaw thrust
Prolonged sedation (eg.: opioids)	Apnea or impaired ventilation	HR $\uparrow$ or $\downarrow$	$ETCO_2$	$\downarrow$ (respiratory acidemia)	Nasal or oral airway
OSA	Cyanosis	RR $\downarrow$			Consider bridging with
	Coarse upper airway sounds	BP $\uparrow$ or $\downarrow$			noninvasive ventilation in
	Snoring	$Spo_2 \downarrow$			appropriate patients[41]
	Paradoxic movement of chest wall and abdomen				Use non-opioid pain management
					Naloxone or flumazenil as indicated
					Reintubation if necessary

Cause	Clinical signs	Vitals	Monitoring	Findings/ABG	Management
Persistent muscle relaxant (~40% of patients have TOF ratio <0.9 in PACU[42])	Floppy, immobile Strength ↓ (head lift, grip) Limited or slurred vocalizations Shallow respirations Use of accessory muscles	T ↔ HR typically ↑ RR typically ↑ (may be ↓ if paralysis is severe) BP typically ↑ SpO_2 ↓	Pulse oximeter $ETCO_2$ TOF/twitch monitor	ABG: PaO_2 ↓, PcO_2 ↑, pH ↓ (respiratory acidemia)	Ensure adequate reversal given Assistive ventilation Reintubation if necessary
Laryngospasm	Absence of breath sounds or severe stridor (if partial obstruction) Paradoxic movement of chest wall and abdomen Copious secretions	T ↔ HR typically ↑, RR ↓, BP typically ↑ SpO_2 ↓	Pulse oximeter $ETCO_2$	Acute condition requiring intervention	Suction to remove stimulus CPAP via a tight fitting mask (in partial obstruction) Forceful jaw thrust Succinylcholine (IV, IM,[43] or submental[44]) and airway management
Secretions (mucus plug), Bleeding, Foreign body	Gurgling Coughing Coarse upper airway sounds May lead to laryngospasm	T ↔ HR typically ↑ RR ↓, ↑ or ↔ BP any SpO_2 ↓	Pulse oximeter $ETCO_2$	Typically nondiagnostic except in the setting of respiratory acidemia	Airway suctioning Ensure all packing, pads, sponges accounted for after oral surgery Excess bleeding may require surgical evaluation

Other causes of airway obstruction in the PACU: bronchospasm, airway edema, trauma, hematoma (external pressure), anaphylaxis.

Abbreviations: ABG, arterial blood gas; ET_{CO_2}, end tidal carbon dioxide; IM, intramuscular.

or suspected OSA, use of a continuous positive airway pressure (CPAP) device can noninvasively improve airway obstruction. These interventions may be unsuccessful, necessitating placement of a laryngeal mask airway or OETT. An endotracheal tube is primarily indicated if supraglottic edema, anaphylaxis (causing airway edema), or bilateral vocal cord paralysis is suspected. *A nasal trumpet is inserted, which alleviates the upper airway obstruction, but BP remains significantly increased from baseline.*

HYPERTENSION

Derangements in BP are common in the postoperative setting. Arterial BP is proximally pulsatile and distally becomes laminar as the pressure gradient diminishes across the arterioles and capillaries. Pulsatile flow is optimal for tissue function and prolonged nonpulsatile flow leads to inadequate tissue perfusion and failure.[4]

BP is expressed as systolic (SBP), diastolic (DBP) and mean arterial pressure (MAP) in mm Hg.

$$MAP = 1/3\,SBP + 2/3\,DBP$$

Pulse pressure (PP) is also commonly used, and may be calculated by:

$$PP = SBP - DBP$$

Systemic vascular resistance (SVR) causes the degradation of pulsatile flow and is a frequently used parameter to quantify vascular tone.

$$SVR = (MAP - central\ venous\ pressure)/CO \times 80$$

SVR depends on 3 variables that must be considered when using it to manage hemodynamic abnormalities.

Hypertension is the sustained elevation of systemic arterial pressure and develops as the resistance in peripheral arteries increases. Left ventricular hypertrophy results from untreated, longstanding hypertension (HTN) and increases O_2 demand, placing the heart at increased risk during any decrease in O_2 supply.[4] Hypertension places patients at risk for cardiovascular disease.[5] Physiologic autoregulation of tissue perfusion may be shifted upwards in patients with HTN.

Causes for HTN in the immediate postoperative period are varied (**Table 5**). Evaluation of HTN initially includes assessment of adequacy of respiratory status and analgesia. Muscle strength and respiratory effort are critical because partially paralyzed, conscious patients often have large increases in BP. Shivering, if present, can increase O_2 consumption by up to 500%, leading to increased respiratory and myocardial demands. Consideration of volume status is essential. Methods to evaluate and monitor volume status are addressed later in this article.

BP monitoring in this situation includes many possibilities. The noninvasive BP (NIBP) cuff is the standard monitor used in the PACU. If HTN is labile or accelerates then a continuous arterial BP monitor is indicated. An intra-arterial catheter (a-line) is the gold standard for continuous direct measurement of BP. Being invasive, it has inherent risks including hematoma formation, infection, embolization, and damage or occlusion of the artery with resultant distal tissue ischemia. With increasing accuracy, emerging alternatives are being used including noninvasive continuous arterial pressure monitoring devices, as described in **Box 2**.

Adequate airway and respiratory status were ensured by administering additional reversal medications. A urinary bladder catheter was inserted and patency of the in situ nasogastric tube (NGT) was confirmed to rule out distention. Non-narcotic

Table 5
Hypertension (the fifth most common PACU complication,[1] occurring in 1.1%–2% of all PACU admissions [SBP>20% of baseline or DBP>110 mm Hg][1,45])

Hypertension

In general:

~30% of the general population more than age 20 y has preexisting hypertension and prevalence increases with age[46]

- Typically occurs in the first 2 h of PACU admission and resolves within a few hours[46]
- Leads to complications including MI, arrhythmias, CHF, pulmonary edema, and stroke[47]
- Increases the risk of hemorrhage after craniotomy[48]

Patients with HTN in the PACU have higher ICU admissions (2.6% vs 0.2%) and mortality (1.9% vs 0.3%) compared with those without this complication[45]

Differential Diagnosis	Clinical Signs and Symptoms	Vital Signs	Monitors	Laboratory Tests	Treatment[47]
Preoperative diagnosis of hypertension	Nonspecific; Documentation in preoperative records	T ↔, HR ↔, RR ↔, BP ↑, Spo2 ↔	NIBP cuff, Arterial line, Noninvasive arterial pressure monitoring	Nonspecific; May have findings related to disease secondary to chronic HTN	Treat underlying causes first: Reduce pain score; Pulmonary support; NGT, Foley, and so forth; Anxiolytics, antipsychotics
Persistent or severe pain	Pain score >4/10; Irritability, agitation; Verbalization; Splinting during respirations	T ↔, HR ↑ or ↔, RR ↑ or ↔, BP ↑, Spo2 ↔	Trend pain scores	Nonspecific	Labetalol: 20 mg initial bolus, 20–80 mg repeat boluses, or start infusion at 1–2 mg/min, maximum 24 h dose 300 mg; Nitroglycerin: 5 μg/min, titrated by 5 μg/min every 5–10 min to maximum of 60 μg/min
Hypoventilation	Cyanosis	T ↔, HR ↑ or ↔, RR any, BP ↑, Spo2 ↓ or ↔	Pulse oximeter ETco2	ABG: many possible abnormalities	Esmolol: 500 μg/kg loading dose over 1 min, infusion at 25–50 μg/kg/min, increase by 25 μg/kg/min every 10–20 min, maximum 300 μg/kg/min; Nicardipine: 5 mg/h, increase 2.5 mg/h increments every 5 min to maximum of 15 mg/h
Hypoxemia	Sedated or cannot be aroused; Snoring, upper airway obstruction; Paradoxic movement of chest wall and abdomen				
Distension of hollow organs (bowel, bladder)	Abdominal fullness; Abdominal distention or pain with palpation; Complaints of constipation or flatulence	T ↔, HR ↑ or ↔, RR typically ↑, BP ↑, Spo2 ↓ or ↔	Bladder ultrasonography	Depending on time course, may reflect postobstructive renal failure	Nitroprusside: 0.5 μg/kg/min, increase to maximum of 2 μg/kg/min; Clevidipine: 2 mg/h, double every 3 min to effect, maximum 132 mg/h
Anxiety Delirium	Clinical findings consistent with confusion, disorientation, feelings of impending doom, or other derangements	T ↔, HR ↑ or ↔, RR ↑ or ↔, BP ↑, Spo2 ↓ or ↔	CIWA scale CAM-ICU score	Nonspecific	Intermittent bolus therapy with metoprolol and hydralazine are widely used in practice to treat PACU HTN

Other causes of acute hypertension in the PACU: shivering, hypervolemia, increased ICP, inappropriate monitors (eg.: wrong size cuff, misplaced transducer).

Abbreviations: CHF, congestive heart failure; ICP, intracranial pressure; ICU, intensive care unit; N/V, nausea and vomiting.

Box 2
Noninvasive continuous arterial pressure monitoring devices

BP changes in patients following GA, and especially in the immediate postoperative period, can be rapid and extreme. The gold standard for the measurement of BP historically has been the intra-arterial catheter; however, this device can lead to significant complications including arterial injury, air embolism, and even limb ischemia. Because continuous BP monitoring is frequently indicated for patients with significant systemic disease, new methods of noninvasive continuous arterial pressure monitoring have been developed in recent years. Devices reported in the literature include CNAP,[6] Colin tonometer,[7] Finapres,[8] Nexfin,[9,10] and Tensys TL-200.[11] Although the specific advantages and disadvantages of each individual device are beyond the scope of this article, the following information is typical of the various devices within this group:

- The devices record noninvasive arterial pressure via radial artery compression/decompression,[11] finger photoplethysmography,[10] or the volume-clamp finger cuff method[6,9]

- Differences between noninvasive measurements and intra-arterial measurements vary significantly between devices and studies, with a wide range of accuracy or inaccuracy

- Devices are limited in use when distal upper extremity arterial flow is dampened or compromised

- Most devices rely on distal to proximal pressure reconstruction and waveform filtering, which is an indirect measure of arterial pressure

Devices for the noninvasive measurement of arterial blood pressure have been in development for many years; however, to date, accuracy and intraoperative reliability vary widely. With recent advancements, these devices seem to offer a reasonable alternative in patients in whom intra-arterial catheterization is not strictly indicated but noninvasive blood pressure cuff use and accuracy is limited by clinical or patient-specific confounding factors. These devices are not indicated in critically ill patients or unstable patients.

---

analgesics were administered based on her OSA history and somnolence. A b-blocker was administered because the patient was taking one before surgery (she missed several doses with her evolving illness) and because of her current tachycardia. She was not shivering but had a low body temperature measured at 35°C.

HYPOTHERMIA

Hypothermia is a recognized perioperative risk requiring preemptive intervention. Mechanisms for heat loss include radiation, conduction, convection, respiration, and evaporation.[12] A core body temperature less than 36°C is classified as perioperative hypothermia. The physiologic effects of hypothermia (**Table 6**) depend on the temperature level and duration of exposure.

Hypothermia is a risk after surgery because of increased heat loss with vasodilation under GA, increased exposed body surface area, administration of cool intravenous fluids, and low room temperatures. The implications of hypothermia on perioperative hemodynamics include increased SVR, myocardial irritability, and susceptibility to arrhythmias. Coagulopathy, another complication of hypothermia can exacerbate hypovolemia in patients with postoperative hemorrhage. Temperature is typically monitored during surgery and strategies to maintain normothermia are used including forced air warmers, fluid warmers, adjusting ambient room temperature, and warming mattresses (**Table 7**). Hypothermia may decrease metabolism of medications and interfere with muscle relaxant reversal, prolonging their effects. Multiple devices using

Table 6
Physiologic effects of hypothermia

Effect	Comment
Shivering	↑ O_2 consumption up to 500%
Coagulopathy	Reversible with rewarming
Immunosuppression	Increased wound infections
Arrhythmias	Tachycardia → bradycardia
Diuresis with resultant electrolyte abnormalities	Hypokalemia, hypomagnesemia, and hypophosphatemia
↑ cardiac output	—
HTN	—
Vasoconstriction	—

Data from Aslam AF, Aslam AK, Vasavada BC, et al. Hypothermia: evaluation, electrocardiographic manifestations, and management. Am J Med 2006;119(4):297–301.

a variety of methods have been used to determine postoperative temperature including infrared-based devices measuring tympanic or temporal artery temperatures. Continuous monitoring can be accomplished using skin, oral, rectal, bladder, and blood sensors. Case reports of a newer technology indicated for temperature monitoring controlled hypothermia, the endovascular temperature regulation catheter, may be useful in the future. The endovascular catheter has all the inherent risks of invasive central lines but the added advantage of rapid and precise temperature control and continuous monitoring (**Box 3**).

A forced air warming device was used to treat hypothermia. The patient remained minimally responsive despite ensuring adequate oxygenation, ventilation, muscle relaxant reversal, and hemodynamics. After treating airway obstruction, hypertension,

Table 7
Treatment of hypothermia

	Methods of Rewarming	Rewarming (°C/h)
Passive external	Blankets	0.5–4
	Humidified inspired air	Variable
Active external	Forced warmed air	1–2.5
	Warm blankets	Variable
	Warm water immersion	2–4
Active internal	Warm humidified air	0.5–1.2
	Warm intravenous fluids	Variable
	Body cavity lavage	Variable
	Endovascular rewarming	1.5–3
Extracorporeal	Hemodialysis, hemofiltration	2–3
	Cardiopulmonary bypass	7–10

Data from Longo DL, Fauci AS, Kasper DL, et al. Chapter 19. Hypothermia and frostbite. In: Longo DL, Fauci AS, Kasper DL, et al, editors. Harrison's principles of internal medicine. 18th edition. New York: McGraw-Hill; 2012.

> **Box 3**
> **Postoperative hypothermia**
>
> Maintaining core body temperature in patients undergoing surgery and requiring anesthesia has become an important topic in the literature. Surgery, especially in the setting of general, regional, or neuraxial anesthesia, puts patients at risk for postoperative hypothermia and related complications, posing significant danger. A study by Hines and colleagues[1] prospectively evaluating 18,473 consecutive patients in PACUs found that:
>
> - If initial temperature (tympanic membrane) was less than 35°C, PACU stay was 152 ± 46 minutes
> - If temperature was between 35°C and 36°C, PACU stay was 129 ± 60 minutes
> - If temperature was greater than or equal to 36°C, PACU stay was 111 ± 65 minutes
>
> Hypothermia is typically defined as a core body temperature less than 36°C, with severe hypothermia defined as a core temperature of less than 28°C.

and hypothermia, her vital signs were: BP, 140/85 mm Hg; T, 35C; RR, 24. The patient's HR trended downward, ultimately to 29 bpm.

SINUS BRADYCARDIA

HR fluctuations are common during surgery. The sinus node normally controls HR in a consistent range and is responsive to physiologic challenges and derangements. The normal HR is 60 to 100 bpm and is optimal for adequate cardiac output, tissue perfusion, and myocardial oxygenation. However, the unique nature of coronary blood flow makes HR an important consideration when abnormal. Coronary blood flow in the left ventricle (LV) occurs almost exclusively during diastole because of increased pressures generated by LV contraction, which leaves the LV more vulnerable to ischemia, especially if coronary atherosclerosis and left ventricular hypertrophy are present. The lower-pressure right ventricle generally has perfusion throughout the cardiac cycle.

Factors that decrease coronary perfusion include decreased diastolic BP, increased LV end diastolic pressure, and tachycardia. Diastole is shortened more than systole during tachycardia, resulting in a significant decrease in coronary perfusion to the LV. Imbalanced myocardial O_2 supply and demand frequently lead to myocardial ischemia. There is little myocardial O_2 reserve because of the high O_2 extraction by myocardial tissue.[13] (Physiologic effects of sinus bradycardia (SB) and sinus tachycardia (ST) are listed in **Table 8**.)

Bradycardia in the perioperative period can have both beneficial and detrimental effects on hemodynamics. Keeping HR low is necessary for high-risk patients with CAD to minimize myocardial ischemia by decreasing O_2 demand while increasing

Table 8 Hemodynamic effects of sinus rhythm abnormalities	
Sinus Bradycardia	**Sinus Tachycardia**
↓ cardiac output (caused by ↓ HR)	↓ cardiac output (caused by ↓ SV)
Hypotension	Hypotension
Syncope	Syncope
Asystole	Myocardial ischemia

supply.[14] However, the POISE,[15] trial showed that expanding β blocker use to patients at low risk for myocardial ischemia had an increased incidence of complications including stroke. In addition, because HR is one of the primary determinants of cardiac output, bradycardia in a patient who is unable to increase myocardial contractility or SV may experience hypotension and inadequate cardiac output.

Bradycardia immediately following GA is frequently caused by the muscarinic effects of acetylcholinesterase inhibitors used for the reversal of nondepolarizing muscle relaxants. Although less common, bradycardia resulting from myocardial ischemia or hypoxia is more concerning. High-grade or complete heart block may rarely present as bradycardia in the perioperative period. Medications that slow HR (**Table 9**) can also contribute, as in this scenario.

Evaluation of bradycardia should include vital signs (ensuring adequate respiratory status, Spo_2, and BP), the timing of medication administration, and a 12-lead electrocardiogram (ECG). Defibrillator patches connected to an external pacing device can be applied if medical management fails to resolve the bradycardia, and this may be followed by judicious administration of an anticholinerergic such as atropine or glycopyrrolate to increase HR. If there is no pharmacologic response and the BP is low or unstable, transcutaneous pacing can be instituted. The external pacemaker should be set for an appropriate rate between 80 and 100 bpm and amplitude should be adjusted to a level 10% higher than the pacing threshold. Significant patient discomfort can be expected with this procedure and appropriate sedation is recommended.

A transvenous temporary pacing catheter is also an option if transcutaneous pacing is unsuccessful. However, transvenous pacing requires central venous access and the

Table 9
Bradycardia or sinus tachycardia (dysrhythmia is the fourth most common PACU complication,[1] occurring in 1.4% of all PACU admissions)

Bradycardia or sinus trachycardia		
Sinus Tachycardia: Differential Diagnosis		**Treatment**
Anemia	Electrolyte abnormalities	1. Identify and correct or treat the underlying cause
MI	Fever/sepsis	
Medications	Pulmonary embolism	2. If the patient is young and otherwise healthy, permissive tachycardia as an appropriate response can be monitored without intervention
Hypoxia	Anxiety	
Hypovolemia	Malignant hyperthermia	
Pain	Pheochromocytoma	
Hypercarbia	Thyrotoxicosis	3. Rate control
Acidemia		
Bradycardia: Differential Diagnosis		**Treatment**
MI	Medications:	1. Identify and correct or treat the underlying cause
Heart block	β-Blockers	
Increased ICP	Calcium channel blockers	2. If the patient is otherwise hemodynamically stable and the HR is >40–45 bpm, consider close monitoring only
OSA	Amiodarone	
Hypothermia	Digoxin	
Epidural anesthesia	Anticholinesterase inhibitors	3. Atropine, glycopyrrolate, glucagon (not FDA approved)
Surgical irritation	Narcotics	
	Propofol	4. Transcutaneous pacing, transvenous pacing, or medications (isoproterenol)
	Dexmedetomidine	

Abbreviation: FDA, US Food and Drug Administration.

lead can be difficult to position and secure for reliable capture and pacing, which may cause a delay in therapy for those unfamiliar with its use.

After ensuring adequate oxygenation, ventilation, and BP (now 95/48 mmHg), external pacing patches were applied and atropine was administered because of its rapid onset and the degree of bradycardia present. A 12-lead ECG did not reveal ischemic changes. The patient responded appropriately with these interventions and her HR increased to 137 bpm. The HR was persistently increased throughout the next hour.

SINUS TACHYCARDIA

Tachycardia's effects on perioperative hemodynamics, like bradycardia, may be beneficial or harmful. Persistent tachycardia increases myocardial O_2 demand and limits supply, thereby increasing the risk of ischemia. However, cardiac output may be supported by mild tachycardia in certain patients. Tachycardia may also indicate perioperative hypovolemia, hemorrhage, hyperglycemia, and increased metabolic demand.

Ensuring adequate pain control, intravascular volume, oxygenation, and ventilation are the first steps to treating ST. Determining the Hb is also warranted if acute hemorrhage is suspected. Vagolytic effects from the reversal of muscle relaxants are also common and require no treatment unless there are concerns for myocardial ischemia. Management of ST primarily depends on the accurate diagnosis and treatment of the underlying cause.

On the monitor, the patient displayed ST, which was initially treated with a fluid bolus after ensuring adequate analgesia and ruling out hypoxia and hypercarbia. The Hb was determined using a point of care device and found to be 9 g/dL. There was no response to these interventions, her HR further increased, and her rhythm became irregular.

ATRIAL FIBRILLATION

Atrial fibrillation (A-Fib) is common, with a frequency of approximately 0.4% in the general population, and is most prevalent in caucasians, men, and patients more than 60 years of age.[16] Risk factors include congestive heart failure (CHF), HTN, and CAD. A-Fib produces an irregular rhythm on ECG tracing based on fibrillation of the atria with inconsistent impulse conduction through the atrioventricular node. Hemodynamic consequences of A-Fib relate to the loss of atrial kick and rapid ventricular HR (**Box 4**). Atrial kick typically delivers 15% additional volume to the ventricle before systole and can contribute as much as 40% during exercise. Loss of this

---

Box 4
Hemodynamic effects of A-Fib

↓ cardiac output (↓ preload)

Myocardial ischemia

Hypotension

Syncope

Ventricular tachycardia

Cardiomyopathy

additional preload affects cardiac output, especially in patients with increased LV end diastolic pressures or decreased LV compliance. Rapid ventricular response causes increased coronary O_2 demand while decreasing supply because of the reduction in the diastolic component of the cardiac cycle.[16]

A-Fib occasionally presents in the PACU. This abnormal rhythm can have profound effects on the perioperative hemodynamic profile of patients (**Table 10**). Supraventricular rhythms are the most common aberration and are often manifest by a decreased BP and cardiac output.[16] They are more easily managed and have more stable hemodynamic pictures than ventricular arrhythmias. Although less common, ventricular arrhythmias are more concerning and require aggressive intervention including synchronized cardioversion (CDVN) or defibrillation. These abnormal rhythms may result from increased catecholamines from surgical stress, hemorrhage, fluid shifts, electrolyte abnormalities, hypoxia, hypercarbia, myocardial ischemia, or conduction abnormalities.

Continuous ECG is essential for ongoing monitoring, and a 12-lead ECG is needed for diagnosis. Placement of defibrillator patches assists with monitoring and intervention. Hemoglobin determination is essential as well as inspection of the surgical site to rule out hemorrhage. Other laboratory studies including an electrolyte panel or arterial blood gas may suggest the cause. Correction of hypoxia, hypercarbia, and electrolyte abnormalities is indicated. Controlling the HR is essential to avoid myocardial ischemia, especially in patients with underlying CAD. Adenosine can be therapeutic in the case of SVT or diagnostic in the case of A-Fib with rapid ventricular response. In all cases of arrhythmias, synchronized CDVN or defibrillation is indicated if the patient becomes hemodynamically unstable. However, this may only be transiently successful if the underlying cause of the arrhythmia is not corrected.

A 12-lead ECG was obtained that showed A-Fib with a rapid ventricular response. STand T-wave changes were present in the inferior leads, indicating myocardial stress or ischemia. Metoprolol was given to control HR. Blood pressure remained marginal and SpO2 was stable. HR decreased but the patient remained in A-Fib with a rate of 110 bpm. Amiodarone was considered but withheld because of marginal BP that continued to decline over the next 45 minutes.

HYPOTENSION

Perioperative hypotension occurs in approximately 2.7% of patients in the PACU.[1] The potential causes of prolonged hypotension are diverse, but the risk of inadequate tissue perfusion has a common end point: shock. Tissue hypoperfusion (O_2 supply and demand imbalance) results in impaired organ function, anaerobic metabolism with lactic acidosis, and neuroendocrine and inflammatory responses. The shift to anaerobic metabolism produces excess lactic acid, which presents as an increased load to the liver for conversion.[17]

Compensatory mechanisms are geared toward preserving cerebral and coronary perfusion. Activation of the sympathetic nervous system occurs with varying degrees of hemodynamic response depending on the degree of hypoperfusion (**Box 5**). Initial stages of shock are usually reversible with appropriate resuscitation but, if left untreated, become unresponsive to therapy.[18] Recommendations for optimal MAP vary in hemodynamically unstable patients with hemorrhagic shock (40 mm Hg), traumatic brain injury (90 mm Hg), and others (65 mm Hg).[19,20]

Hypotension has implications for all organ systems and requires immediate investigation and intervention. Although many causes exist (**Table 11**), common causes include residual drug effects (which are less likely as the time from

Table 10
Atrial fibrillation (dysrhythmia is the fourth most common PACU complication,[1] occurring in 1.4% of all PACU admissions)

A-Fib

In general:
New onset A-Fib in postoperative noncardiothoracic patients has an incidence of ~0.4%[49,50]
Patients developing A-Fib are typically older and undergoing emergency procedures[50]
Risk ratio for overall mortality is 1.7–1.8 times that for patients without A-Fib[51]

Differential Diagnosis	Clinical Signs and Symptoms	Vital Signs	Monitors	Laboratory Tests	Treatment
MI	Pale, diaphoretic; New onset or changed murmur (especially mitral regurgitation); Jugular venous distension; Wheezing or cough	T ↔, maybe ↑; HR ↑ or ↓; RR typically ↑; BP usually ↑; SpO2 ↓ or ↔	ECG (continuous and 12 lead); Echo; Arterial pressure monitoring?	Troponin, CK-MB	1. Identify and correct or treat the underlying cause. 2. If the patient is unstable and the rhythm is clearly A-Fib, consider urgent cardioversion. 3. If the patient is otherwise stable, control the ventricular response rate and attempt pharmacologic conversion (if less than 48 h from onset) a. Amiodarone has a conversion rate of 13%–42%[52,53] but a relapse rate of up to 55%[54] b. Metoprolol has a quoted conversion rate of ~40%[55]. 4. If patients remain in A-Fib, anticoagulation may be indicated. Typical recommendations[55] for postoperative rate control in patients developing A-Fib (with no contraindications) include: First line: β-blockers. Second line: diltiazem or verapamil. Amiodarone and digoxin are not widely recommended for rate control in A-Fib following surgery
Anemia	Pale, vasoconstricted; Lethargy; Orthostatic hypotension	T ↔; HR ↑; RR ↑ or ↔; BP typically ↓; SpO2 ↓ or ↔	Examine surgical site and drains; POC Hb	CBC; Coagulation studies (if continued bleeding)	
Increased sympathetic activity (Hyperthermia, exposure to adrenergic agents)	Patient may appear normal, anxious, or obtunded; In patients with hyperthermia, findings may be consistent with sepsis	T typically ↑; HR ↑; RR typically ↑; BP ↑ or ↓; SpO2 ↓ or ↔	HR monitoring; Temperature monitoring	Nonspecific	
Pulmonary edema; Pulmonary hypertension	Frothy white or pink sputum; Rales or rhonchi on auscultation; Loud S2 (pulmonic valve closure); Sternal heaving, use of accessory muscles, dyspnea	T ↔; HR typically ↑; RR ↑; BP ↑; SpO2 typically ↓	Consider CXR	ABG: PaO2 typically ↓, PCO2 any, pH any	
Electrolyte abnormalities (especially potassium and magnesium)	Peaked T-waves (↑ K+) or T-wave flattening or inversion (↓ K+) on ECG; Findings consistent with electrolyte imbalances	T ↔; HR typically ↑; RR any; BP any; SpO2 ↔	Nonspecific; Continuous ECG during extreme electrolyte imbalance	Basic chemistry panel	

Other causes of A-Fib in the PACU: hypoxia, hypervolemia, hypovolemia.

Abbreviations: CXR, chest radiograph; POC, point of care.

Box 5
Hemodynamic effects of hypotension

↑ Vasomotor tone

↑ HR

↑ Contractility

---

administration increases), hypovolemia, acute hemorrhage, cardiac insufficiency or arrhythmias, and metabolic derangements. Aggressive efforts must be undertaken to determine the cause of postoperative hypotension and to intervene to avoid further decline. For example, amiodarone is an effective agent for HR control and potential conversion of A-Fib to SR but can lead to hypotension with initial bolus.

Laboratory studies to investigate the cause of hypotension include blood gas analysis, troponin I, CBC, and BMP. The ST and T-wave changes noted on the previous ECG raise the index of suspicion for myocardial ischemia, and determination of volume status, cardiac output, and cardiac index are necessary (especially in this patient with a history of ICM and CAD). Invasive lines (central venous pressure [CVP] and pulmonary artery catheters [PAC]) are commonly used and rely on pressure to estimate cardiac preload volumes. Newer, noninvasive cardiac output devices are being used with increasing frequency (**Box 6**), especially because the usefulness of PACs has been called into question.[21] Transthoracic echocardiography (TTE) or transesophageal echocardiography (TEE) is also helpful in this instance to evaluate wall motion abnormalities, valvular function, and ventricular filling. A newer TEE device (ImaCorTM) allows probe placement, cardiac evaluation, and an option to leave the probe in situ safely or to remove and save it for reinsertion up to 72 hours later. More research and experience is needed to delineate the role of this device in postoperative care. A chest radiograph is indicated to evaluate for pulmonary disorders or if central access is placed. A diagnosis of pneumothorax, pulmonary embolism, and cardiac tamponade also should be entertained.

An a-line was placed for continuous BP monitoring. The evaluation of hypotension revealed possible myocardial ischemia (TEE showed decreased LV function) so the continuous TEE probe was removed and saved. A-Fib converted back to ST after administering a slow bolus of amiodarone with subsequent continuous infusion. The Hct had decreased by 15% following additional crystalloid boluses, but the abdomen was becoming distended and firm (NGT was functional). The coagulation indices worsened revealing a mild coagulopathy, and T decreased to 34.8°C despite forced air warming efforts. Blood pressure improved with conversion to SR, volume resuscitation, and a norepinephrine infusion, but then urine output was decreased.

OLIGURIA

Oliguria in the postoperative period is potentially a sensitive indicator of hemodynamic adequacy for several reasons. Oliguria may reflect hemodynamic derangements that need further investigation and management. Hypovolemia (prerenal state) is the most common cause, although attention to the classic causes surrounding hypoperfusion, renal injury (acute, chronic, or acute on chronic), and postrenal causes must be considered (**Table 12**).

Table 11
Hypotension (the third most common PACU complication,[1] occurring in 2.2%–2.7% of all PACU admissions[1,45] [SBP <20% of baseline for >15 minutes])

Hypotension

In general[45]:

Postoperative hypotensive episodes mostly depend on surgical factors (vs patient characteristics or anesthetic choice)

- Surgical time increases the risk of postoperative hypotension (less than 1 h vs greater than 1 h)
- Ear, nose, and throat; gynecology; and general intra-abdominal surgical procedures may have a higher risk of postoperative hypotension

Patients noted to have intraoperative hypotension are at higher risk for postoperative hypotension

Differential Diagnosis	Clinical Signs and Symptoms	Vital Signs	Monitors	Laboratory Tests	Treatment
Inadequate fluid replacement Hemorrhage/anemia	Dark, concentrated urine Decreased urine output Orthostatic changes in blood pressure Increased respiratory variation in pulse oximeter, CVP or arterial line tracings	T ↔ HR ↑ RR ↑ or ↔ BP ↓ Spo$_2$ typically ↔	NIBP cuff Arterial line Noninvasive Arterial pressure monitoring CVP Urinary catheter	CBC or point of care testing will reveal acute anemia	~80% of patients can be managed with volume alone (crystalloid, colloid or blood products)[1] ~20% of patients require pressors or other intervention[1]
Cardiogenic hypotension (MI, low cardiac output or CHF, cardiac tamponade, pulmonary embolus)	Consistent with underlying mechanism Generally cool, dry, pale extremities reflecting poor peripheral blood flow In acute MI, patients may be diaphoretic	T typically ↔ HR any but likely ↑ RR ↑ or ↔ BP ↓ Spo$_2$ ↓ or ↔	As listed earlier plus: ECG PA catheter Echo Noninvasive cardiac output monitoring	Troponin, CK-MB	Rule out life threatening conditions first Cautious volume resuscitation as dictated by monitors Support blood pressure with pressors as needed to maintain organ profusion Consider cardiology or cardiac surgery consultation as needs dictate

Arrhythmias	Palpitations Irregular heart rate Syncope Angina Dizziness	T ↔ HR any RR ↑ or ↔ BP ↓ or ↑ SpO_2 ↓ or ↔	As listed earlier plus: ECG (continuous and 12 lead)	Troponin, CK-MB if concern for ischemia	Cardioversion for any acutely destabilizing arrhythmia Rate control and/or conversion of A-Fib or flutter Rate control for ST
Septic shock Hypoadrenalism Vasoplegia Anaphylaxis	Evaluate preoperative cultures and medications Examine urimeter for signs of UTI Evaluate intraoperative and postoperative exposures (medications, latex, adhesives, and so forth)	T any but likely ↑ HR usually ↑ RR ↑ BP ↓ SpO_2 ↓ or ↔	NIBP cuff Arterial line Noninvasive arterial pressure monitoring CVP Urinary catheter	Nonspecific Cortisol measurements may be nondiagnostic	Maintain end-organ perfusion with volume resuscitation and pressors Treatment of anaphylaxis includes: 100% Fio_2, epinephrine, IVFs, β-adrenergics, anticholinergics, steroids, and antihistamines[56] Methylene blue has been used to treat some forms of vasoplegia[57]
Pneumothorax Excessive PEEP	Decreased breath sounds (with pneumothorax) Cause may be recent placement of a central line Sensation of dyspnea with excess PEEP	T ↔ HR ↑ RR ↑ BP ↓ SpO_2 ↓ or ↔	CXR Examine chest tubes and sites for air leaks	Nonspecific	Reduce PEEP and increase maneuvers to otherwise improve oxygenation as needed Pneumothorax may require placement of a chest tube

Other causes of hypotension in the PACU: medications, superior vena cava syndrome, acidemia, electrolyte derangement, sympathectomy (neuraxial).

Abbreviations: PEEP, positive end-expiratory pressure; UTI, urinary tract infection.

Box 6
Minimally invasive/noninvasive cardiac output monitoring

The current gold standard for monitoring of cardiac output is the pulmonary artery catheter (PAC). This device, described most famously by Swan and colleagues,[22] has proved to be an acceptable measure of cardiac output and central pressures, but its use has not definitively improved postoperative patient care in the literature.[21] Furthermore, the PAC has been associated with major adverse events including infection, arrhythmias, and rupture of the pulmonary artery.[23] Over time, devices to replace the PAC in a minimally invasive or noninvasive manner have been developed using varied methods such as arterial pulse contour analysis, esophageal Doppler, lithium dilution, thoracic bioimpedance, and other novel techniques.

Arterial pulse contour analysis: These devices measure changes in systolic pressure between inspiration and expiration during mechanical ventilation, which can be extrapolated to define volume status in appropriate patients.[24,25]

Esophageal Doppler: These devices measure velocity in the descending aorta using the assumption that the aorta is a cylinder, multiplying area by velocity to define flow and, further, stroke volume (by defining area under the curve of pulsatile flow over time).[26]

Dilution techniques: The initial dilution techniques described in the literature used indocyanine green; however, more recent devices use lithium as an indicator. In current use, a low-dose bolus of lithium chloride is injected intravenously and lithium concentration decay is measured over time. This decay versus time graph can then describe cardiac output based on area under the curve.[26]

Thoracic bioimpedance: This technique is the least invasive of the common alternative cardiac output measurement devices. This method measures electrical resistance between electrodes on the upper and lower thorax, which is proportional to total intrathoracic fluid volume. This measurement and the change in values are then used to describe cardiac output via changes in total bioimpedance.

Advantages and disadvantages of the various methods are as follows:

Method	Advantages	Disadvantages
Arterial pulse contour analysis	Arterial line only	More invasive than some measures
	Continuous cardiac output measured	Requires a quality, undampened arterial tracing
	Can measure stroke volume	May need recalibration during large hemodynamic swings
Esophageal Doppler	Simple to use	Requires some assumptions about unmeasured variables
	No circulatory access required	Does not measure flow in the aortic arch (upper extremities, head)
	In use since the 1970s, well understood	Requires some operator learning
	Similar in size to a nasogastric tube	
Dilution techniques	Easy to set up	Requires circulatory access
	Arterial line only	Requires multiple blood draws
	Continuous cardiac output measured	Interference caused by neuromuscular blocking drugs
	Can measure stroke volume	Does not adequately define preload

Thoracic bioimpedance	No invasive monitoring required of any kind	Requires skilled setup
		Requires some assumptions about unmeasured variables
		Not useful in patients with arrhythmias
		Limited use in the presence of interference from operating room devices

Data from Funk DJ, Moretti EW, Gan TJ. Minimally invasive cardiac output monitoring in the perioperative setting. Anesth Analg. 2009;108(3):887–7.

Evaluation should begin with assessing for postrenal obstruction. Irrigation of an in situ urinary bladder catheter assesses patency of the urinary collecting system including the bladder and urethra. This assessment does not guarantee obstruction-free passage of urine from the renal collecting system to the bladder via the ureters. If the patient does not have a urinary catheter, one should be placed to continuously measure urine output. Bladder volume can also be assessed with an ultrasound-based bladder scanner. Optimization of hemodynamics and volume status is essential to support adequate renal perfusion. The laboratory studies previously undertaken contribute to the assessment of the urgency and necessity for more aggressive interventions (e.g.: treatment of hyperkalemia and acidosis).

In addition, consideration must be given to intra-abdominal hypertension (IAH) and abdominal compartment syndrome (ACS) in patients with tight fascial closures, intra-abdominal hemorrhage, large volume resuscitation, or bowel ischemia. When a patient presents with a distended, firm abdomen and oliguria, measurement of bladder pressures is indicated. Sustained pressures greater than 20 mm Hg with organ dysfunction define the presence of ACS.[27] There are commercially available devices to facilitate measurement of bladder pressure and they can be useful as ongoing monitors (**Box 7**).

Fluid challenges were given and volume optimization was achieved with the use of a noninvasive cardiac output device. Hematocrit was stable, but her abdomen was firm. Bladder pressures were normal (no ACS) and cardiac output was decreased from baseline. Her CR subsequently measured 3.2 (from a baseline of 1.6) with a potassium of 4.6 mmol/L. The norepinephrine infusion was continued and an epinephrine infusion was started to increase cardiac output. The hemodynamics improved, but she remained hypothermic. Her respiratory status was adequate.

Despite continuous care, monitoring, and aggressive intervention, she became progressively more lethargic, hypoxic and hypercarbic, hypertensive, coagulopathic, anemic, and hypothermic. She was intubated, further resuscitated, and transferred to the surgical intensive care unit for continued management of her presumed sepsis.

The appearance of oliguria in this scenario is expected. This patient is experiencing multiple hemodynamic problems that can affect renal blood flow and perfusion. She has a firm, distended abdomen after recent abdominal surgery (potentially caused by bleeding), intestinal edema from ischemia (with hypotension), and volume expansion. She also has preexisting renal dysfunction which makes her more susceptible to insults, especially after the administration of radiocontrast before surgery. There are no specific renal protective interventions other than supporting hemodynamics, BP, and renal perfusion. If she has increased bladder pressures, reoperation to alleviate the potential abdominal compartment syndrome is indicated.[27]

Table 12
Oliguria (occurs in 0.8% of patients having noncardiac surgery in first 7 days after surgery[58], postoperative urinary retention varies from 5% to 70%[59])

Oliguria
Generally defined as less than 0.3–0.5 mL/kg/h or less than 300–500 mL/d

Differential Diagnosis	Clinical Signs and Symptoms	Vital Signs	Monitors	Laboratory Tests	Treatment
Hypovolemia (bleeding, sepsis, inadequate intraoperative resuscitation)	Altered mental status Dry mucous membranes Diminished skin turgor Increased respiratory variation in pulse oximeter, CVP, or arterial line tracings	T any HR ↑ RR ↑ or ↔ BP ↓ Spo$_2$ ↔	Urinary catheter Examine surgical site and drains	CBC Urine electrolytes (↓ UNa, ↑ UOsm, FENa <1%)	Maintain end-organ perfusion with volume resuscitation and pressors ~80% of patients can be managed with volume alone (crystalloid, colloid, or blood products)[1] ~20% of patients require pressors or other intervention[1]
Decreased renal blood flow (hypotension, IAH, low cardiac output, renal artery obstruction, aortic dissection)	Signs and symptoms associated with a low cardiac output state or cardiogenic shock Abdominal discomfort or distension in IAH/ACS Discordant blood pressure in the upper extremities in dissection	T ↔ HR ↑ RR ↑ or ↔ BP any Spo$_2$ ↔	Urinary catheter Bladder pressure May require more invasive monitors such as an arterial line, CVP, PA catheter	Urine electrolytes (↓ UNa, ↑ UOsm, FENa <1%)	Support cardiac output and blood pressure with cautious fluid resuscitation and pressors as indicated Assess for signs of life threatening surgical complications Consultation with advanced diagnostic teams (cardiothoracic surgery, radiology, vascular surgery)
Baseline renal dysfunction	Review patient chart Important not to forget that patients with poor	T ↔ HR ↔ RR ↔	Urinary catheter	Increased baseline creatinine/BUN	Supportive care, maintaining adequate renal perfusion

	preoperative function are at higher risk after surgery	BP ↔ Spo₂ ↔				
Radiocontrast media	Recent exposure to contrast: Vascular surgery Cardiac endovascular procedures Neuroangiography Recent CT scan		Nonspecific	Urinary catheter	Nonspecific Late increase in serum creatinine/BUN	Preexposure therapy with[60]: 1. Discontinue diuretics and NSAIDs before the procedure if possible 2. 150 mEq sodium bicarbonate in 1 L of D5W IV at 1 mL/kg per hour for 6–12 h before the procedure 3. N-acetylcysteine 600 or 1200 mg by mouth twice a day on the day before and day of the procedure Postexposure: supportive care, IVF
Postrenal causes (ureter, bladder, or urethral injury/block; catheter dysfunction)	History of BPH or nephrolithiasis Following injury during intra-abdominal procedures (especially obstetrics/gynecology, urology, or general surgery procedures)	T ↔ HR ↑ or ↔ RR ↑ or ↔ BP ↑ or ↔ Spo₂ ↓ or ↔		Urinary catheter as indicated	Nonspecific Late increase in serum creatinine/BUN	Check indwelling urinary catheters for obstruction or malfunction

Other causes of oliguria in the PACU: medications (e.g.: anticholinergics, renal toxicity), neuraxial anesthesia, acute tubular necrosis, SIADH

Abbreviations: BUN, blood urea nitrogen; NSAIDs, nonsteroidal antiinflammatory drugs; SIADH, syndrome of inappropriate antidiuretic hormone.

Box 7
Bladder pressure monitoring

Increased intra-abdominal pressure (IAP) in the perioperative period can lead to IAH and ACS, increasing morbidity and mortality.[28] Although the incidence of reported ACS varies in the literature between 1%[29] and 14%,[28] or more in at-risk patients, even among intensive care–trained physicians, nearly 1 in 4 are unfamiliar with bladder pressure monitoring.[30] Contraindications to bladder pressure monitoring are similar to those for placement of a transurethral catheter: recent history of bladder surgery, hematuria, unexplored pelvic trauma, or neurogenic bladder.

ACS occurs in a wide variety of patient settings, including trauma,[31] severe burns (generally greater than 40%–50% of body surface area),[32,33] severe intra-abdominal disorders or aggravation (liver transplantation, pancreatitis, massive intra-abdominal bleeding, or other conditions),[34] sepsis,[35] and conditions involving large fluid shifts or volume resuscitation, encompassing perioperative patients.

Risk factors for IAH/ACS (adapted from Ref.[27]):

- Reduced abdominal wall compliance
  - Acute respiratory failure with increased intrathoracic pressure
  - Abdominal surgery with tight closures
  - Surgery in the prone position
  - Patients with an increased BMI
- Increased intraluminal contents or gastrointestinal obstruction
- Ascites or increased intra-abdominal contents
- Capillary leak or fluid resuscitation
  - Acidosis (pH <7.2)
  - Hypothermia (temperature <33°C)
  - Massive transfusion (>10 units of blood in 24 hours)
  - Coagulopathy (platelet count <55000/mm^3, PT >15 seconds, PTT >2 times normal, or INR >1.5)
  - Massive fluid resuscitation (>5L/24 hours)
  - Pancreatitis
  - Sepsis

Consensus recommendations from the World Society of the Abdominal Compartment Syndrome (WSACS)[27,36] include (1) early serial IAP monitoring in patients at risk, (2) enhancing abdominal wall compliance, (3) evacuating intraluminal contents, (4) evacuating abdominal fluid collections, (5) correcting positive fluid balance, (6) acutely managing end-organ perfusion, and (7) surgical intervention as indicated by clinical monitoring.

If a patient has 2 or more risk factors for IAH/ACS in the presence of progressive organ failure, the WSACS recommends measuring a patient's IAP to establish a baseline pressure. IAP should be measured via bladder pressure and[27]:

1. Expressed in mm Hg
2. Measured at end expiration
3. Performed in the supine position
4. Zeroed in the midaxillary line
5. Performed with instillation volume of 25 mL of saline or less
6. Measured 30 to 60 seconds after instillation (allows bladder relaxation to occur)
7. Measured when abdominal muscles are relaxed

Pressures should be measured every 4 hours or more frequently. A sustained pressure greater than or equal to 12 mm Hg represents IAH, whereas a pressure greater than or equal to 20 mm Hg with new organ failure suggests ACS. Commercial devices currently available for the measurement of bladder pressure are similar in design and include the AbViser AutoValve, the Bard Intra-abdominal Pressure Monitoring Device, and the Holtech Foley Manometer.

REFERENCES

1. Hines R, Barash PG, Watrous G, et al. Complications occurring in the postanesthesia care unit: a survey. Anesth Analg 1992;74(4):503–9.
2. Standards for basic anesthetic monitoring. Approved by the ASA House of Delegates on October 21, 1986, and last amended on October 20, 2010 with an effective date of July 1, 2011. Available at: http://www.asahq-org/for-members/standards-guidelines-and-statements.aspx.
3. Eichhorn JH. Prevention of intraoperative anesthesia accidents and related severe injury through safety monitoring. Anesthesiology 1989;70(4):572–7.
4. Barrett KE, Barman SM, Boitano S, et al. Chapter 31. Blood as a circulatory fluid & the dynamics of blood & lymph flow. In: Barrett KE, Barman SM, Boitano S, et al, editors. Ganong's review of medical physiology. 24th edition. New York: McGraw-Hill; 2012. Available at: http://www.accessmedicine.com/content.aspx?aID=56264612. Accessed July 30, 2012.
5. Ogedegbe G, Pickering TG. Chapter 68. Epidemiology of hypertension. In: Fuster V, Walsh RA, Harrington RA, editors. Hurst's the heart. 13th edition. New York: McGraw-Hill; 2011. Available at: http://www.accessmedicine.com/content.aspx?aID=7823628. Accessed July 30, 2012.
6. McCarthy T, Telec N, Dennis A, et al. Ability of non-invasive intermittent blood pressure monitoring and a continuous non-invasive arterial pressure monitor (CNAP™) to provide new readings in each 1-min interval during elective caesarean section under spinal anaesthesia. Anaesthesia 2012;67(3):274–9.
7. Steiner LA, Johnston AJ, Salvador R, et al. Validation of a tonometric noninvasive arterial blood pressure monitor in the intensive care setting. Anaesthesia 2003;58(5):448–54.
8. Smith SM, Samani NJ, Sammons EL, et al. Influence of non-invasive measurements of arterial blood pressure in frequency and time-domain estimates of cardiac baroreflex sensitivity. J Hypertens 2008;26(1):76–82.
9. Martina JR, Westerhof BE, van Goudoever J, et al. Noninvasive continuous arterial blood pressure monitoring with Nexfin®. Anesthesiology 2012;116(5):1092–103.
10. Fischer MO, Avram R, Cârjaliu I, et al. Non-invasive continuous arterial pressure and cardiac index monitoring with Nexfin after cardiac surgery. Br J Anaesth 2012. advance access. [Epub ahead of print].
11. Dueck R, Goedje O, Clopton P. Noninvasive continuous beat-to-beat radial artery pressure via TL-200 applanation tonometry. J Clin Monit Comput 2012;26(2):75–83.
12. Longo DL, Fauci AS, Kasper DL, et al. Chapter 19. Hypothermia and frostbite. In: Longo DL, Fauci AS, Kasper DL, et al, editors. Harrison's principles of internal medicine. 18th edition. New York: McGraw-Hill; 2012. Available at: http://www.accessmedicine.com/content.aspx?aID=9095933. Accessed July 30, 2012.
13. Morgan GE Jr, Mikhail MS, Murray MJ. Chapter 19. Cardiovascular physiology & anesthesia. In: Morgan GE Jr, Mikhail MS, Murray MJ, editors. Clinical anesthesiology. 4th edition. New York: McGraw-Hill; 2006. Available at: http://www.accessmedicine.com/content.aspx?aID=889833. Accessed July 30, 2012.
14. Mangano DT, Layug EL, Wallace A, et al. Effect of atenolol on mortality and cardiovascular morbidity after noncardiac surgery. Multicenter Study of Perioperative Ischemia Research Group. N Engl J Med 1996;335(23):1713–20.
15. Devereaux PJ, Yang H, Yusuf S, et al. Effects of extended-release metoprolol succinate in patients undergoing non-cardiac surgery (POISE trial): a randomised controlled trial. Lancet 2008;371(9627):1839–47.

16. Prystowsky EN, Padanilam BJ, Waldo AL. Chapter 40. Atrial fibrillation, atrial flutter, and atrial tachycardia. In: Fuster V, Walsh RA, Harrington RA, editors. Hurst's the heart. 13th edition. New York: McGraw-Hill; 2011. Available at: http://www.accessmedicine.com/content.aspx?aID=7813732. Accessed July 30, 2012.

17. German MS. Chapter 17. Pancreatic hormones and diabetes mellitus. In: Gardner DG, Shoback D, editors. Greenspan's basic & clinical endocrinology. 9th edition. New York: McGraw-Hill; 2011. Available at: http://www.accessmedicine.com/content.aspx?aID=8407307. Accessed July 30, 2012.

18. Zuckerbraun BS, Peitzman AB, Billiar TR. Chapter 5. Shock. In: Brunicardi FC, Andersen DK, Billiar TR, et al, editors. Schwartz's principles of surgery. 9th edition. New York: McGraw-Hill; 2010. Available at: http://www.accessmedicine.com/content.aspx?aID=5011953. Accessed July 30, 2012.

19. Nguyen HB, Huang DT, Pinsky MR. Chapter 34. Hemodynamic monitoring. In: Tintinalli JE, Stapczynski JS, Cline DM, et al, editors. Tintinalli's emergency medicine: a comprehensive study guide. 7th edition. New York: McGraw-Hill; 2011. Available at: http://www.accessmedicine.com/content.aspx?aID=6370270. Accessed July 30, 2012.

20. Antonelli M, Levy M, Andrews PJ, et al. Hemodynamic monitoring in shock and implications for management. International Consensus Conference, Paris, France, 27–28 April 2006. Intensive Care Med 2007;33(4):575–90.

21. Connors AF, Speroff T, Dawson NV, et al. The effectiveness of right heart catheterization in the initial care of critically III patients. JAMA 1996;276(11):889–97.

22. Swan HJ, Ganz W, Forrester J, et al. Catheterization of the heart in man with use of a flow-directed balloon-tipped catheter. N Engl J Med 1970;283(9):447–51.

23. Domino KB, Bowdle TA, Posner KL, et al. Injuries and liability related to central vascular catheters: a closed claims analysis. Anesthesiology 2004;100(6):1411–8.

24. Michard F, Boussat S, Chemla D, et al. Relation between respiratory changes in arterial pulse pressure and fluid responsiveness in septic patients with acute circulatory failure. Am J Respir Crit Care Med 2000;162(1):134–8.

25. Michard F. Changes in arterial pressure during mechanical ventilation. Anesthesiology 2005;103(2):419–28.

26. Funk DJ, Moretti EW, Gan TJ. Minimally invasive cardiac output monitoring in the perioperative setting. Anesth Analg 2009;108(3):887–97.

27. Cheatham ML, Malbrain ML, Kirkpatrick A, et al. Results from the International Conference of Experts on Intra-abdominal Hypertension and Abdominal Compartment Syndrome. II. Recommendations. Intensive Care Med 2007;33(6):951–62.

28. Balogh Z, Mckinley BA, Holcomb JB, et al. Both primary and secondary abdominal compartment syndrome can be predicted early and are harbingers of multiple organ failure. J Trauma 2003;54(5):848–59.

29. Hong JJ, Cohn SM, Perez JM, et al. Prospective study of the incidence and outcome of intra-abdominal hypertension and the abdominal compartment syndrome. Br J Surg 2002;89(5):591–6.

30. Kimball EJ, Rollins MD, Mone MC, et al. Survey of intensive care physicians on the recognition and management of intra-abdominal hypertension and abdominal compartment syndrome. Crit Care Med 2006;34(9):2340–8.

31. Ertel W, Oberholzer A, Platz A, et al. Incidence and clinical pattern of the abdominal compartment syndrome after "damage-control" laparotomy in 311 patients with severe abdominal and/or pelvic trauma. Crit Care Med 2000;28(6):1747–53.

32. Markell KW, Renz EM, White CE, et al. Abdominal complications after severe burns. J Am Coll Surg 2009;208(5):940–7.
33. Hershberger RC, Hunt JL, Arnoldo BD, et al. Abdominal compartment syndrome in the severely burned patient. J Burn Care Res 2007;28(5):708–14.
34. Santa-Teresa P, Muñoz J, Montero I, et al. Incidence and prognosis of intra-abdominal hypertension in critically ill medical patients: a prospective epidemiological study. Ann Intensive Care 2012;2(Suppl 1):S3.
35. Regueira T, Bruhn A, Hasbun P, et al. Intra-abdominal hypertension: incidence and association with organ dysfunction during early septic shock. J Crit Care 2008;23(4):461–7.
36. Cheatham ML, Safcsak K. Is the evolving management of intra-abdominal hypertension and abdominal compartment syndrome improving survival? Crit Care Med 2010;38(2):402–7.
37. Patel PM, Patel HH, Roth DM. Chapter 19. General anesthetics and therapeutic gases. In: Brunton LL, Chabner BA, Knollmann BC, editors. Goodman & Gilman's the pharmacological basis of therapeutics. 12th edition. New York: McGraw-Hill; 2011. Available at: http://www.accessmedicine.com/content.aspx?aID=16664636. Accessed July 30, 2012.
38. Marshall BE, Wyche MQ. Hypoxemia during and after anesthesia. Anesthesiology 1972;37(2):178–209.
39. Mathew JP, Rosenbaum SH, O'Connor T, et al. Emergency tracheal intubation in the postanesthesia care unit: physician error or patient disease? Anesth Analg 1990;71(6):691–7.
40. Ramachandran SK, Nafiu OO, Ghaferi A, et al. Independent predictors and outcomes of unanticipated early postoperative tracheal intubation after nonemergent, noncardiac surgery. Anesthesiology 2011;115(1):44–53.
41. Jaber S, Chanques G, Jung B. Postoperative noninvasive ventilation. Anesthesiology 2010;112(2):453–61.
42. Murphy GS, Brull SJ. Residual neuromuscular block: lessons unlearned. Part I: definitions, incidence, and adverse physiologic effects of residual neuromuscular block. Anesth Analg 2010;111(1):120–8.
43. Landsman IS. Mechanisms and treatment of laryngospasm. Int Anesthesiol Clin 1997;35(3):67–73.
44. Redden RJ, Miller M, Campbell RL. Submental administration of succinylcholine in children. Anesth Prog 1990;37(6):296–300.
45. Rose DK, Cohen MM, Deboer DP. Cardiovascular events in the postanesthesia care unit: contribution of risk factors. Anesthesiology 1996;84(4):772–81.
46. Hajjar I, Kotchen TA. Trends in prevalence, awareness, treatment, and control of hypertension in the United States, 1988–2000. JAMA 2003;290(2):199–206.
47. Marik PE, Varon J. Perioperative hypertension: a review of current and emerging therapeutic agents. J Clin Anesth 2009;21(3):220–9.
48. Basali A, Mascha EJ, Kalfas I, et al. Relation between perioperative hypertension and intracranial hemorrhage after craniotomy. Anesthesiology 2000;93(1):48–54.
49. Christians KK, Wu B, Quebbeman EJ, et al. Postoperative atrial fibrillation in non-cardiothoracic surgical patients. Am J Surg 2001;182(6):713–5.
50. Sohn GH, Shin DH, Byun KM, et al. The incidence and predictors of postoperative atrial fibrillation after noncardiothoracic surgery. Korean Circ J 2009;39(3):100–4.
51. Coumel P. Paroxysmal atrial fibrillation: a disorder of autonomic tone? Eur Heart J 1994;15(Suppl A):9–16.

52. McAlister HF, Luke RA, Whitlock RM, et al. Intravenous amiodarone bolus versus oral quinidine for atrial flutter and fibrillation after cardiac operations. J Thorac Cardiovasc Surg 1990;99(5):911–8.

53. Larbuisson R, Venneman I, Stiels B. The efficacy and safety of intravenous propafenone versus intravenous amiodarone in the conversion of atrial fibrillation or flutter after cardiac surgery. J Cardiothorac Vasc Anesth 1996;10(2):229–34.

54. Di Biasi P, Scrofani R, Paje A, et al. Intravenous amiodarone vs propafenone for atrial fibrillation and flutter after cardiac operation. Eur J Cardiothorac Surg 1995; 9(10):587–91.

55. Martinez EA, Epstein AE, Bass EB. Pharmacologic control of ventricular rate: American College of Chest Physicians guidelines for the prevention and management of postoperative atrial fibrillation after cardiac surgery. Chest 2005;128(Suppl 2): 56S–60S.

56. Hepner DL, Castells MC. Anaphylaxis during the perioperative period. Anesth Analg 2003;97(5):1381–95.

57. Leyh RG, Kofidis T, Strüber M, et al. Methylene blue: the drug of choice for catecholamine-refractory vasoplegia after cardiopulmonary bypass? J Thorac Cardiovasc Surg 2003;125(6):1426–31.

58. Kheterpal S, Tremper KK, Englesbe MJ, et al. Predictors of postoperative acute renal failure after noncardiac surgery in patients with previously normal renal function. Anesthesiology 2007;107(6):892–902.

59. Baldini G, Bagry H, Aprikian A, et al. Postoperative urinary retention: anesthetic and perioperative considerations. Anesthesiology 2009;110(5):1139–57.

60. Gleeson TG, Bulugahapitiya S. Contrast-induced nephropathy. AJR Am J Roentgenol 2004;183(6):1673–89.

Perioperative Quality and Improvement

Richard Morrow, MBA, MBB

KEYWORDS

- Plan, Do, Study, Act • Perioperative quality • Surgical Care Improvement Project
- Lean Six Sigma

KEY POINTS

- Measurement is important in increasing quality improvement.
- Teams in perioperative services will do well in their improvement efforts by learning and using Lean and Six Sigma PDSA (Plan, Do, Study, Act) methodologies.
- Perioperative quality starts with having clearly defined roles, responsibilities, and tasks in safety practices.
- Standard work is essentially composed of 3 elements: (1) the right work: the right way to do a task; (2) the right sequence; (3) the right time.

A CASE FOR QUALITY IMPROVEMENT

Health care quality and safety are becoming more transparent, and consumers will increasingly value a health care organization's (HCO) safety and quality rating in choosing where they go for surgery. The HCOs whose perioperative teams learn and apply quality improvement skills and help their organization improve such ratings faster than their competitors will also be more financially secure. Perioperative services are major drivers to a hospital's safety rating because of the dominance of surgical safety measures in the Centers for Medicare and Medicaid Services (CMS) Accountable Care Value-Based Purchasing Score[1] and a recent Consumer Reports hospital safety report.[2] Surgical services are often the most, or one of the most, profitable services, and loss of referrals and poor media reports will directly reduce margins.

In its August 2012 inaugural hospital safety report announcement, Consumer Reports shares with readers, "Infections, surgical mistakes, and other medical harm contribute to the deaths of 180,000 hospital patients a year, according to projections based on a 2010 report from the Department of Health and Human Services. Another 1.4 million are seriously hurt by their hospital care." This Consumer Reports publication states these mistakes are only from Medicare patients' experiences. The report

Quality, Safety, Reliability, Healthcare Performance Partners, Nashville, TN, USA
E-mail address: rmorrow@hpp.bz

Anesthesiology Clin 30 (2012) 555–563
http://dx.doi.org/10.1016/j.anclin.2012.07.011   anesthesiology.theclinics.com
1932-2275/12/$ – see front matter © 2012 Elsevier Inc. All rights reserved.

shares that it is only reporting on fewer than 20% of the hospitals, because hospitals either choose that it is not important enough to report or are not required to report. Patients may have negative reactions to hospitals and health systems who avoid reporting.

The airline and automotive industries have publicly reported quality and safety for years. There is little doubt that consumers use these measures in their purchase decisions. Health care and surgical services will be no exception to this trend. This article's purpose is to guide leaders and perioperative staff in how to start improving perioperative quality and safety.

LEAD WITH MEASURE

Measurement is important in increasing quality improvement. More than 10% of patients undergoing colorectal surgeries experience an infection.[3] Three percent or more of patients who receive a coronary artery bypass graft (CABG) acquire an infection within the area of the chest or organ space.[4] Some major academic medical centers report CABG surgical-site infections (SSIs) 2 to 3 times higher than this rate. There are practices known to reduce the risk of infection, and organizations embracing quality assurance have improved virtually every Surgical Care Improvement Project (SCIP) measure,[5] including the choice and timing of a prophylactic antibiotic. This goal was accomplished using quality improvement methods discussed in this article. Yet many perioperative teams fail to train themselves in scientific improvement methodologies and in achieving compliance to these guidelines.

PENN MEDICINE IMPROVES COMPLIANCE

One example of an organization embracing improvement is the University of Pennsylvania Health System. These teams found the contributing factors in explaining failures in administering the antibiotic at the right time. The teams used Penn Medicine's Performance Improvement In Action (PIIA) problem-solving methodology, based on Lean, Six Sigma, and Change Leadership, to achieve a higher compliance. The teams learned this scientific methodology and applied measurement to understand the issue, analyze contributing factors, and judge the effectiveness of countermeasures. After achieving a level of compliance, they maintained measurement to control and sustain the gains in complying in the timing of antibiotics before surgery. Compliance of 100% is possible, as these teams discovered and proved.

IMPROVEMENT METHODOLOGIES

The steps gone through by the aforementioned team are often described as Six Sigma's Define, Measure, Analyze, Improve, and Control, with the acronym DMAIC. Six Sigma was developed by Motorola[6] to solve its quality issues back in the 1980s when it was losing market share and profitability because of poor quality. Motorola turned its quality around, crediting its Six Sigma, and became one of the first winners of the Malcolm Baldrige Award for quality. Six Sigma's roots go back to the 1920s when Shewhart and Deming pioneered scientific methodologies for team problem solving, and named their steps "Plan, Do. Study (Check), and Act" with the acronyms PDSA and PDCA. Only PDSA is used here for simplicity.

Lean is another common term in health care improvement, and is based on PDSA with an emphasis on reducing waste. Toyota is credited with developing a quality improvement methodology it calls the Toyota Production System, a foundation of Lean. Six Sigma, Lean, and PDSA are consistent with each other and are the most common methodologies in health care today. Teams in perioperative services will do well in their improvement efforts by learning and using these methodologies. One may refer to these methodologies as "recipes" for teams to follow in improvement efforts.

CHANGE LEADERSHIP MUST BE ADDED TO THE RECIPE

Change leadership refers to the practice of engaging people in the problem-solving effort. The need to help people in change cannot be overemphasized. Some organizations use the term change management for a similar purpose. However, change management is a poor term for what is required. Morrow[7] argues that change "leadership" is a better term for when improvement is needed. Change management is perhaps a better term for sustaining a change once the desired performance is achieved.

FIRST, AND NOT LEAST, LEADERSHIP'S ROLE IN QUALITY IMPROVEMENT

Leadership is key to making these recipes result in great "meals." The cook and recipe at dinner are analogous to a leader and problem-solving methodology in perioperative quality improvement. The greatest recipe on earth will not result in a good meal if the cook fails to follow the recipe. A leader not following the problem-solving methodology will risk the team's ability in enjoying improvement.

Health care organizations need to train leaders in how to lead change as much as to train teams in problem-solving methodology. Dr Mark Chassin, President of The Joint Commission, and the author ensured that his Robust Process Improvement (RPI) scientific methodology using the author's Lean and Six Sigma included leadership training first. Executive leadership and the team leaders' direct manager were taught their roles and how to support teams, and the need to follow the RPI methodology. This program continues to be used in solving some of health care's most vexing issues including surgical safety. The author has used Lean, Six Sigma, and Change Leadership to reduce the risk of wrong-site surgery, and results to date include zero wrong-site surgery since 2008 in one health care system.[8] A scientific methodology with strong leadership is key to improving perioperative quality and safety.

A LESSON IN NOT FOLLOWING THE RECIPE IN PERIOPERATIVE IMPROVEMENT

Sometimes we learn better by failing. In this case study, I (R.M.) was asked to mentor a team leader in perioperative services charged with reducing SSIs. The team leader was trained in Six Sigma and change management. The organization's leadership told me before I started that their earlier Six Sigma program failed, and described projects as "moving at a glacial pace." It did not take me long to realize the reason.

The first step in any scientific methodology is to define clearly the sponsor and her or his measures of success. A charter I developed years ago[7] is a step-by-step approach in ensuring the sponsor and team leaders are in synchronization with the issue and measures of success. This charter includes goals, scope, names of process owners, core team members who will meet frequently with the team leaders and deploy the methodology, names of other key stakeholders, and a project plan with timeline of report backs to the sponsor.

I should have known this project was in trouble when the Executive Sponsor asked for the signed charter and found that after a month into the project the team leader had yet to accomplish getting signatures from the sponsor or any member. Teams should have an understandable charter signed by the sponsor and posted for all to see. Engaging the perioperative staff and seeing a leader's signature is a good test of clarity and is a sign of leadership commitment. Four months later the team leader had yet to accomplish this task. This team struggled on several fronts simply from not following these scientific methodologies.

Next on the failure list is a frequent issue among teams that struggle to rapidly improve a process. The second phase of Six Sigma is Measure, which requires a timely measure of the key outcome. Excuses abounded from the team leader and others as to why SSIs could not be reported daily or within 2 months of the date of procedure. As a further sign measurement was needed, I had surgeons exclaim surprise when I shared with them the SSI rate. It was clear that the outcomes were not measured well enough because measurement and transparency of the measure were not in place. A team that fails to measure the key outcomes followed soon after with process measures that correlate with outcomes will struggle. So, please, "bite the bullet" in getting measures posted early and the pain will be much less (Sorry about the play on words, anesthesiologists.)

FOLLOWING A ROAD MAP TO GUIDE PERIOPERATIVE QUALITY IMPROVEMENT MAKES PROBLEM SOLVING EASIER

Many problem-solving teams have a road map that includes steps to guide a team through its methodology. There is one for DMAIC at www.rpmexec.com. Such road maps guide the team and help them not miss steps, such as signed charters and posting measurements. There are many successes when the Define and Measure phases are done well, as in the Penn Medicine success. Penn Medicine continues to succeed in improving its perioperative quality through its PIIA.

It must also be realized that before teams were trained in how to solve problems using a road map, leaders were trained in the foundation of performance improvement. Leaders were taught their roles and an overview of their improvement methodology before teams were engaged. The Penn leaders expect to sign charters followed by a baseline measure of the outcomes soon after. These tasks are also noted on the better road maps.

CASE STUDY ON SURGICAL SAFETY IMPROVEMENT: THE TIME-OUT

Anyone who has witnessed surgical "time-outs" has experienced good ones and bad ones. A time-out is a key feature of surgical safety and is required in many countries. A good time-out is one whereby every team member pauses and becomes aware that the correct patient is on the table and the surgeon's intentions are confirmed, detailing both site and procedure immediately before incision or entry.

All too often the time-out is called by a nurse and the time-out is hurried, with only a few paying attention. In far too many cases the operating surgeon may not even be in the room. In all the years of investigating wrong-site, wrong-side, and wrong-procedure events, the author has never found that the nurse is the one who cut on the wrong patient, the wrong site, or did the wrong procedure. So why are these surgical team members often the only ones listening and performing a pause?

Perioperative quality starts with having clearly defined roles, responsibilities, and tasks in safety practices. Standard work is key to quality and is as important, if not more important in surgery, because of its complexity and ever-changing situations and variables. Standard work is essentially composed of 3 elements:

1. The right work: the right way to do a task
2. The right sequence
3. The right time. The right time includes an ability of meeting the time required to meet the customer's demand. SSIs are correlated with time of procedure, and

anything that delays the procedure should be avoided. Health care workers trained in Lean know this as meeting takt time. Takt time shows the time at which each process step must be performed to meet the demand of the patient or customer.

A valuable use of standard work in perioperative services is in performing a time-out. There are only 3 elements required in a time-out, and doing it correctly often can be improved by eliminating work in a time-out that should be done elsewhere. The author often hears a check of allergies in a time-out. If surgeons complain of time-outs taking too long, perhaps the time-out is taking too long. Maybe there are too many questions being asked during the time-out. The question about allergies should be moved to earlier in the perioperative process when the allergy question is most important, thus reserving the critical time-out work to focus the team on validating the correct patient identity, site, and procedure. Quality improvement efforts often result in less time required to do the task well.

JOB AIDS

Components of standard work may include job aids, which are clear and easy-to-read task lists and often checklists, and are in the workplace, immediately and conveniently available (not in a binder on a dusty shelf). Perioperative teams may have standard work, but they also need to use that concept of measure again to get the most out of their efforts to create a quality process.

Compliance to the standard work is to be measured and assessed by the staff and their managers periodically, with coaching done in the moment. Measuring the performance of the perioperative team in their standard work is a must. Many perioperative teams never measure the compliance to the time-out. In one organization where improved time-outs were implemented, not the fact that the time-out was performed but how well the time-out was performed was measured. In other words, the culture was changed to one that made the team members feel uncomfortable not doing a time-out. Once that was achieved, the number of attempts to get everyone to stop and pay attention was measured. In other words, the measurement system was matured to drive continuous improvement. Now, the team was measuring not if the time-out occurred, but how easy was it to start and the culture in the room. Again, quality does not take more time. We all can relate to non–value-added tasks required by regulators and accrediting organizations. Once a process is stable and capable of meeting requirements and is mistake-proofed or fail-safed, the next variable can be measured.

Measurement of performance is key in improving quality and safety. Doing a time-out misses the point if the effort is not sincere. A team will do well if they start their problem-solving efforts by observing each role in the perioperative process and how well the tasks are being done. In time-outs, probably the most talked about checklist in perioperative services, One must make sure the team is focused intently on the patient, site marking, and surgeon confirming intent, and make it easy for the team to accomplish.

KEEP JOB AIDS SIMPLE AND USE TECHNOLOGY THAT IMPROVES, NOT DETRACTS FROM, QUALITY

One hospital was "techno savvy" with its time-out checklist. It invested in large flat-screen monitors in every operating room (OR), and trained nurses on how to pull up their version of the time-out on the screen. Initially I (R.M.) thought this was very neat because the circulating nurse would scroll through the questions, guiding the time-out conversation. When I observed their procedures, however, I found everyone

---

Box 1
The Joint Commission's universal protocol for preventing wrong surgery, wrong procedure, and wrong-person surgery

CONDUCT A PREPROCEDURE VERIFICATION PROCESS

Address missing information or discrepancies before starting the procedure

- Verify the correct procedure, for the correct patient, at the correct site.
- When possible, involve the patient in the verification process.
- Identify the items that must be available for the procedure.
- Use a standardized list to verify the availability of items for the procedure. (It is not necessary to document that the list was used for each patient.) At a minimum, these items include:
  - Relevant documentation examples: history and physical, signed consent form, preanesthesia assessment
  - Labeled diagnostic and radiology test results that are properly displayed. Examples: radiology images and scans, pathology reports, biopsy reports
  - Any required blood products, implants, devices, special equipment
- Match the items that are to be available in the procedure area to the patient.

MARK THE PROCEDURE SITE

At a minimum, mark the site when there is more than one possible location for the procedure and when performing the procedure in a different location could harm the patient.

- The site does not need to be marked for bilateral structures. Examples: tonsils, ovaries.
- For spinal procedures: Mark the general spinal region on the skin. Special intraoperative imaging techniques may be used to locate and mark the exact vertebral level.
- Mark the site before the procedure is performed.
- If possible, involve the patient in the site-marking process.
- The site is marked by a licensed independent practitioner who is ultimately accountable for the procedure and will be present when the procedure is performed.[a]
- Ultimately, the licensed independent practitioner is accountable for the procedure, even when delegating site marking.
- The mark is unambiguous and is used consistently throughout the organization.
- The mark is made at or near the procedure site.
- The mark is sufficiently permanent to be visible after skin preparation and draping.
- Adhesive markers are not the sole means of marking the site.
- For patients who refuse site marking or when it is technically or anatomically impossible or impractical to mark the site (see examples below), use your organization's written, alternative process to ensure that the correct site is operated on. Examples of situations that involve alternative processes:
  - Mucosal surfaces or perineum
  - Minimal-access procedures treating a lateralized internal organ, whether percutaneous or through a natural orifice
  - Teeth
  - Premature infants, for whom the mark may cause a permanent tattoo

PERFORM A TIME-OUT

The procedure is not started until all questions or concerns are resolved.

- Conduct a time-out immediately before starting the invasive procedure or making the incision.

- A designated member of the team starts the time-out.

- The time-out is standardized.

- The time-out involves the immediate members of the procedure team: the individual performing the procedure, anesthesia providers, circulating nurse, OR technician, and other active participants who will be participating in the procedure from the beginning.

- All relevant members of the procedure team actively communicate during the time-out.

- During the time-out, the team members agree, at a minimum, on the following:

  ○ Correct patient identity

  ○ Correct site

  ○ Procedure to be done

- When the same patient has 2 or more procedures: If the person performing the procedure changes, another time-out needs to be performed before starting each procedure.

- Document the completion of the time-out. The organization determines the amount and type of documentation.

[a] In limited circumstances, site marking may be delegated to some medical residents, physician assistants (PA), or advanced practice registered nurses (APRN).

Adapted from the full Universal Protocol. For specific requirements of the Universal Protocol, see The Joint Commission standards. Available at: http://www.jointcommission.org/assets/1/18/UP_Poster1.PDF.

looking at the screen with no one looking at the site mark or patient. Is this like texting while driving? One must be careful to not have technology become the focal point, especially when used for quality inspections, as this takes the team members' focus away from the work.

I like to see the surgeon and one other scrubbed person literally point and touch the site mark for all to see physically the intention of the surgeon. I learned this safety technique in operations whereby attaching the wrong component could result in catastrophic failure, and while observing airline pilots pointing to the altitude-setting dial while reading a checklist or reading back what a controller commanded.

We all know that checklists and readbacks can be mundane. To stay alert to the instructions, more focus may be needed to ensure the altitude setting really was what the controller wanted. Pointing and touching are very natural to us. Try this little experiment to see how we naturally want to point to confirm to others. At lunch next time, ask the person across from you where his or her fork or drink is. Watch what he or she does. Use this easy focusing tool in health care whenever you want some extra assurance that the team is paying attention.

ANESTHESIOLOGISTS ARE KEY TO IMPROVING PERIOPERATIVE QUALITY IMPROVEMENT

The Chief of Anesthesiology at a major academic medical center shared this insight with me. Anesthesiologists have a unique advantage in improving surgical quality and safety. Surgeons may see only a few of their colleagues in the course of a day in surgery, but anesthesiologists often work in the ORs with many different surgeons and surgical teams. Anesthesiologists see many good practices that they often share with other surgeons and teams, and they see their fair share of practices that vary and need quality improvement.

Anesthesiologist Applying Lean Six Sigma

At Mount Sinai Medical Center in New York City, Dr Amanda Rhee, Assistant Professor of Anesthesiology, is using her knowledge of clinical practices to maximize the value of Six Sigma approaches to understanding gaps in compliance with antibiotic administration protocols that are enhancements to SCIP measures.

Dr Rhee followed the road map, and this led to decisions on where to focus improvement efforts in enhancing compliance, with the goal of reducing complications. She and her team identified variations in timing and administration of antibiotics and are working on reducing this variation, especially in higher-risk patients. Hypothesis testing and confidence-interval comparisons provide encouragement that their problem-solving approach and identification of variables will make improvements more effectively and quickly.

In many surgical safety issues, such as wrong patient events and SSI, the occurrence of failure is very low and observation alone is unlikely to result in understanding the process issues as quickly as using data analysis and observation. Thus, perioperative teams in quality improvement need a good mix of observation and data-analysis skills. Teams also need to know how to "swarm" the issues as they are occurring and to not rely on observational data alone.

SUMMARY

Perioperative quality and improvement are key to many hospitals' strategic plan, reputation, and margin, because of the risk of poor quality and safety. Transparency in quality, especially in perioperative services, is becoming much greater with CMS' Value-Based Purchasing measures, more media attention on medical errors, consumer groups demanding more transparency, and increased awareness by patients and family of others who have experienced medical errors and poor quality. Payers will likely jump on the CMS bandwagon, and reinforce favorably those who have the highest quality and penalize those who do not (**Box 1**).

Perioperative teams and HCOs that improve in safety and achieve higher safety will reduce cost. Better yet, these HCOs could actually leverage their improvements by increasing their volume and margin as other health care organizations fail to address safety and slip in ratings. In other words, those who improve will improve at a great rate because of the increase in transparency of those who are not improving.

REFERENCES

1. Administration implements new health reform provision to improve care quality, lower costs. Available at: http://www.healthcare.gov/news/factsheets/2011/04/valuebasedpurchasing04292011a.html. Published April 29, 2011. Accessed July 5, 2012.
2. How safe is your hospital? http://www.consumerreports.org/cro/magazine/2012/08/how-safe-is-your-hospital/index.html.
3. Konishi T, Watanabe T, Kishimoto J, et al. Elective colon and rectal surgery differ in risk factors for wound infection. Ann Surg 2006;244(5):758–63.
4. Available at: http://www.nuhcs.com.sg/about-us/clinical-outcomes/coronary-artery-bypass-graft-cabg-infection.html.

5. Surgical Care Improvement Project. February 2011. Available at: http://www.joint commission.org/surgical_care_improvement_project/. Accessed July 22, 2012.
6. "What is Six Sigma?" Motorola University Training Document. Available at: http:// www.motorola.com/web/Business/_Moto_University/_Documents/_Static_Files/ What_is_SixSigma.pdf. Accessed July 22, 2012.
7. Morrow R. Utilizing the 3Ms of process improvement in healthcare: a roadmap to high reliability using lean, six sigma, and change leadership. Boca Raton (FL): CRC Press; 2012.
8. The Wrong Site Surgery Project. Joint Commission Center for Transforming Health-care. Available at: http://www.centerfortransforminghealthcare.org/UserFiles/file/ CTH_Wrong_Site_Surgery_Project_6_24_11.pdf. Accessed July 22, 2012.

Index

Note: Page numbers of article titles are in **boldface** type.

A

Abscess, spinal or epidural, as complication of neuraxial anesthesia, 441

Acute kidney injury, in the PACU, **513–526**
    causes of, 516–519
    definitions, 514–515
    diagnosis in, 522
    epidemiology and risk factors for, 515–516
    management in, 522–523
    presentation of, 521–522
    prevention of, 519–521

Airway obstruction, postoperative, 529–534
    oxygenation, 529–530
    ventilation, 530–534

Anesthesia, neuraxial. See Neuraxial anesthesia.

Anesthesiologists, interdisciplinary rounds in the PACU, **427–431**
    role in perioperative quality improvement, 561–562

Anterior spinal artery syndrome, as complication of neuraxial anesthesia, 440–441

Antiemetics, for postoperative nausea and vomiting, **481–493**
    combinations of, 488
    how to use in practice, 485–487
    prophylaxis with, 482–483
    treatment after prophylaxis, 487–488
    treatment of established, 483–485

Antihistamines, for postoperative nausea and vomiting, 484

Anxiolytics, use in the PACU, **467–480**

Atelectasis, gas-exchange abnormalities under anesthesia, 496
    oxygen and, 496–497

Atrial fibrillation, postoperative, 540–541

B

Back pain, postoperative, with neuraxial anesthesia, 439–440

Bariatric surgery, prophylactic noninvasive ventilation after, 502

Benzodiazepines, anxiolytic use in the PACU, **467–480**

Bilevel positive airway pressure (BiPAP), in the PACU, 498–499

Blood glucose, perioperative. See Glycemic control.

Bradycardia, as complication of neuraxial anesthesia, 440
    postoperative sinus, 538–540

Butyrophenone, for postoperative nausea and vomiting, 484–485

Anesthesiology Clin 30 (2012) 565–571
http://dx.doi.org/10.1016/S1932-2275(12)00103-6
1932-2275/12/$ – see front matter © 2012 Elsevier Inc. All rights reserved.

anesthesiology.theclinics.com

Moving?

Make sure your subscription moves with you!

To notify us of your new address, find your **Clinics Account Number** (located on your mailing label above your name), and contact customer service at:

Email: journalscustomerservice-usa@elsevier.com

800-654-2452 (subscribers in the U.S. & Canada)
314-447-8871 (subscribers outside of the U.S. & Canada)

Fax number: 314-447-8029

Elsevier Health Sciences Division
Subscription Customer Service
3251 Riverport Lane
Maryland Heights, MO 63043

*To ensure uninterrupted delivery of your subscription, please notify us at least 4 weeks in advance of move.

Printed and bound by CPI Group (UK) Ltd, Croydon, CR0 4YY

03/10/2024

01040448-0014